It's Hard to Die!

"Do I Hold On or Do I Let Go?"

❖

Enrique A. Cordero

Email: enrique@eacordero.com
Website: https://www.eacordero.com
Follow: Twitter, Instagram, and Facebook

Interior format by Mary B. Cordero

ISBN-13: 978-1-945812-96-5
Published by Richter Publishing LLC
www.richterpublishing.com
Editor: Haley Morton

Printed in Tampa, Florida, USA.

Cover photo by yupiramos@GoGraph.com
Cover design by Enrique A. Cordero
and Mary B. Cordero

Dedication

This book is dedicated to my Twin Flame, Mary Benedetto Cordero. Your infinite patience, understanding, compassion, spiritual insights, endless words of encouragement, and love that transcends time and space were instrumental in the writing of this book. Thank you for your pearls of wisdom that you provided throughout this entire process.

To my parents, Luis D. Cordero and Maria T. Cordero, for instilling in me an unquenchable thirst for knowledge, a boundless faith, and a spirit of discovery. You taught me to see beyond the obvious. Your presence, guidance, and encouragement have always lifted my spirit and shed light upon my life's journey.

I also dedicate this book to the countless and often nameless men and women in health care: the doctors, nurses, respiratory therapists, laboratory and radiology personnel, patient techs, environmental services (housekeeping), food services, and so many more. These individuals provide the essential functions to those that suffer the vagaries of human existence concerning the physical, mental, emotional, and spiritual upheavals that occur when facing our finitude.

Most importantly, I dedicate this book to all the patients and their families and friends for having taught me so much over the years. You have taught me invaluable lessons that no university can teach. You have all provided me with the ultimate gift, and that is the privilege to learn about life, love, and death.

Acknowledgments

- To my wife, Mary, thank you for your commitment, artistic eye, publishing and copyediting abilities, and the countless sleepless nights that we shared. You have helped bring this publication to fruition.

- To Marianne Posar Duda, MS, RDN, LDN, CNSC, Clinical Nutritionist, thank you for your professional expertise, and for contributing your article, *Artificial Nutrition and Hydration*.

附 80

Disclaimer

The contents of this book are based on over four decades of firsthand experiences, as well as the ideas and opinions of the author. Utmost care has been taken to ensure the accuracy of the information provided. References and information from many diverse sources have been included to encourage you to investigate the subject matter. This book was written to provide you, the reader, with basic facts needed to make informed decisions at the end of life. It is meant to get you to think about this very important subject that we all tend to ignore to one degree or another. The contents of this book do not, in any way, constitute any legal, medical, psychological, religious, or financial advice. The author and publisher are not, in any way, engaged in providing professional health and medical services in this publication. Always consult with your healthcare professionals before making any decisions. The decisions that you make are solely yours.

The author and publisher disclaim any personal or collective liability, directly or indirectly, for the advice or information presented in this book. The anecdotal accounts have been carefully reconstructed to protect the privacy of the individuals. Any similarity to actual cases is purely coincidental.

Introduction

Chapter one of this book is named *So Here I Am—In A Place I Never Imagined*. I will introduce you to a dying patient and his loving wife, Susan. You will witness his devastating illness that forces them to face gut-wrenching end-of-life issues. Were they prepared? What did they do?

I have presented a composite anecdote and intimate portrait of two human beings united in love and facing the ultimate reality of death. Susan and her husband's journeys continue beyond the realm of modern technology associated with death and dying. This narrative includes parts of my own experience and the distressful decisions my wife faced.

Their story continues in my second book, *Now That I Am Dead: What I Should Know At the End of Life*. You will feel Susan's deep unconditional love as she makes her final agonizing decisions that bring bittersweet closure to their loving and spiritual journey.

Why I Wrote this Book

The main purpose of this book is to increase your awareness of this powerful topic, the end of life. It is a subject that is often treated as taboo and, therefore, rarely or superficially discussed until it becomes inevitable. And even then, it is often shrouded and obscured due to fear, pain, and denial. The only way to confront the stark reality of our finitude is to arm ourselves with knowledge and awareness.

Consequently, I have provided you with basic healthcare information and various real-life anecdotes, including my own, to illustrate and shed some light on an otherwise unclear theme. It is my heartfelt wish that the increased awareness and knowledge garnered from this book will help you, someone you love, or your patients make informed decisions at the most crucial point in time, the end of life.

Everyone can benefit from reading this book, regardless of age, faith, ethnicity, or socioeconomic status, including healthcare professionals, because we will all die. Therefore, read, learn, discuss these issues with loved ones, keep this book for the future, and, then, go out and enjoy your life! Live in the here-and-now and look back only to see how far you have traveled on your life's journey. The future is quite tenuous because each step taken today leads you further and further into the future of your own making.

CB EO

C8 80

In the long run, we shape our lives, and we shape ourselves. The process never ends until we die. And the choices we make are ultimately our own responsibility.

Eleanor Roosevelt

Table of Contents

C(3 8)

Death is not extinguishing the light; it is putting out the lamp because dawn has come.

Rabindranath Tagore

CHAPTER ONE

So Here I am—In A Place I Never Imagined

He slowly emerges from the depths and darkness of a sleep of which he has no memory. He starts to become aware of unfamiliar surroundings filled with strange, muffled, and confusing sounds. He feels exposed, naked and helpless; strange people are touching him. Tubes are coming out of every orifice in his body. He has no privacy and no autonomy. He is at the mercy of strangers. They are asking questions that he cannot answer because there is a tube in his mouth. He is groggy, and his eyes cannot focus. His hands are restrained, and as he slowly regains consciousness, he starts to feel relentless pain, discomfort, and extreme dryness in his throat and he starts to think…

Where am I? What happened to me? What's wrong with me? I'm in so much pain I can barely breathe. Who are these damn people holding me down? I can't move! Why are they doing this to me?

Once again, he drifts off into an alien and dark sleep with frown lines on his forehead. Time passes, and once again, he starts to wake up except this time, he is awake much longer and has time to become more aware of his body.

Why do I feel so weak? I'm thirsty. I need water. What is that awful smell? Is it me? What have I done to deserve this? What's wrong with my eyes? They hurt, and I can't see clearly. My head hurts. That sound is driving me crazy! Damn it! STOP sticking me. It hurts! Why the hell can't you understand what I'm saying! Why can't you hear me? Oh, God! I can't breathe! I feel like I'm drowning! Please, God, make it stop! What is that lady doing with those tubes? I feel so cold. Why can't somebody cover me! Where am I? I feel like I'm sinking, can't see, everything ... is ... going ... dark...

He drifts in and out of this twilight world, and eventually, becomes aware of the reality of his situation. It is a reality that is terrifying and one in which he is unable to control. It is a reality which he never envisioned. As he drifts in and out of a drug-induced fog, he loses track of time. Day and night are entwined. It feels surreal, as if time itself has slowed down to a crawl.

How long has it been? I remember that I was sick, but everyone keeps telling me it will be alright. I was home with my family, but I don't remember anything else. What is wrong with me?

I can hear them whispering. What are they saying? Is it about me? Sometimes they come to tell me to 'hang in there,' but I don't feel any better. I am so weak they don't have to hold me down anymore. I can barely open my eyes. I thought I heard...yes! Oh God...that's Susan's voice...my wife! I can't think clearly anymore. I'm tired, so very, very tired...

Eventually, he starts to become aware of the truth. I call it a *knowing*, and it leaves no room for doubt, regardless of what anyone tells you.

Am I going to die? Is this the end? I'm tired of the pain and suffering. I hear everyone around my bed, talking, and sometimes crying. I'm angry because everyone seems to forget that I'm still here. I know they mean well, but I don't want to continue like this. I can't reach out to tell them it's okay and that I will always love them. I'm at peace. They're begging me to stay. I don't want to hurt them, but I'm ready to go. I opened my eyes and was startled! I saw Mom and Dad standing at the foot of my bed. They died years ago. In an instant, they embraced me with their love and offered their hands. There were other people with them, giving off bright light. They looked at me and smiled and then I knew that everything would be fine. We WILL see each other again; I know that this is not the end. I'm not afraid anymore because I know that I'm going to die.

The following anecdote represents some of the bitter turmoil that goes on in the mind of a loved one. In this case, it is the patient's wife, Susan.

Is he going to die? Some tell me there's hope, and others tell me nothing more can be done. Which is it? I want him to live! How can I let him go? I can't believe this is happening! We talked about things like this. We decided that if either one of us were on life support with no chance of surviving, we would let each other go in peace. We promised each other! We promised! Based on unconditional love and trust, we promised each other that we would follow through! Really? This sounds great when you're strong and healthy, but NOW?

Oh, my God! I can't believe this is happening. I don't want him to leave me. I feel sick. I can't eat. I can't sleep. I can't leave his side. I hold his hand, stroke his brow, and kiss him all over his face. I make sure he's clean and cared for properly. I talk to him all the time, and I tell him how much I love him. I know he can hear me. I feel guilty because I secretly beg him every day not to leave me. Then our promise haunts me, and the torment within the deepest recesses of my soul sickens me.

How can I let him go? But I don't want him to suffer! To let him go is painful beyond belief, but to see him suffer like this is excruciating. I know that he wouldn't want to be kept alive in this condition. He's independent, creative, and free. He loves life, and he knows there's more than what our physical senses tell us. What if there's a chance? What if he opens his eyes? What if a miracle occurs? What am I to do? I need to be strong. God, give me strength!

Susan is reluctant to leave her husband's side for fear of what may happen to him if she is not around him. She knows that he can sense her, feel her touch, and hear her words.

I talk to him every single day and tell him how much I love him. I feel so guilty not wanting him to leave me. Am I selfish? We both believe there's more to this life, but if he's gone, I won't be able to kiss him or hold him. I won't hear his laughter, see his smile, or feel his embrace. I won't hear his encouraging words, always supportive, always reassuring. Oh, God, what do I do? I look at him, and it seems as if I'm looking at a stranger. He looks so thin, and I see him gasping for breath through that tube in his mouth. I know that he's medicated. I hope he doesn't feel any pain.

So here I am in a place I never imagined. Even though we discussed these things and promised each other to make the right decision, I am suddenly thrust in front of the ugly face of reality forced to make the 'right' decision! Not all will agree, but I know what he expects of me. My love for him is so profound that I must find the strength to honor our promise, in spite of myself, because I know we'll be together again. I ask for guidance from deep within and reach a resolve. It will be our decision, and we will own it together because we promised.

Here we have an intimate portrait of two human beings united in love and facing the ultimate reality. These anecdotes were created from my countless interactions with critically ill and dying patients, and the conversations with family members, significant others, and friends. Deeply woven into this scenario, I share my personal experience with the readers facing death, and my loving wife has intertwined her most painful choice to keep me on life support, knowing that she might have to reverse her decision.

The characters of Susan and her husband have shared the pain, anguish, uncertainties, despair, concerns, fears, and love with each other. By illustrating what a patient and their loved one experience, I hope to illustrate what facing the possibility of dying feels like to those involved. This information will help you and your family make the best decisions regarding the end of life,

in a timely fashion, so that a peaceful, dignified, and loving end will be experienced.

❖

During the early months of 2001, an unexpected turn of events occurred that would cause a restructuring of my priorities in life. I had never been seriously ill and was in excellent health, biking thirty to fifty miles per week, hiking twenty to twenty-five miles per week, and strength training four times a week. Until, suddenly, I became deathly ill over a short period of two weeks.

I had developed what is called an empyema, which is an accumulation of pus in the pleural space (membranes surrounding the lungs and the chest wall), often resulting from bacterial pneumonia. The mortality rate for this condition can be as high as forty percent to fifty percent. Within twenty-four hours, two chest tubes were inserted, and 1800cc (almost two liters) of pus was drained. I was critically ill and ended up on life support for two weeks. At one point in time, the physicians eventually started to prepare my family for my possible death.

As a healthcare professional familiar with end-of-life issues, I had talked with my wife about this subject, expressing our wishes for such an eventuality. Had my illness turned irreversible, terminal, or without the possibility of a purposeful quality of life, she was prepared to terminate all life-support measures. It was one of those events that most avoid thinking about or one of those incidents that "only happens to other people."

I eventually returned home with an intravenous (IV) pump, since antibiotic therapy needed to continue for another six weeks. Recovery, as you can imagine, was a challenge. Moving a few yards across the room with a walker was an effort, and I was often paralyzed with long bouts of coughing due to the exertion. I was told that it would take a year to recover fully; it took about three months. I was fortunate to have my loving wife by my side, always giving me hope, strength, and loving care. An incredibly loving family and some wonderful caring friends made up the rest of my support circle.

Once I was fully recovered, I returned to my profession as a respiratory therapist. This time, however, with an added perspective that I would use to help my patients and their significant others. I have been keenly familiar with death and dying in my profession, as well as diverse studies that delved into the subject matter. But, having had a brush with death changes the way you look at things, and it makes you think about life and death in a whole different way. It gives you a glimpse of what life should be about and what lies beyond its boundaries.

I am grateful for my experiences and my studies since they have allowed me to help other people far beyond my previous capabilities. My harrowing sojourn as a critically ill patient and my experiences over several decades of caring for terminally ill patients propelled me to write this book.

A Look Behind the Scenes

The greater part of my responsibilities in respiratory therapy have been in the emergency department and the intensive care units. Respiratory therapists form an integral part of the resuscitation team due to our expertise in airway management. Among many other procedures, my responsibilities have included intubation (inserting a breathing tube into the trachea, or windpipe), extubation (removal of the breathing tube), terminal extubations (death is expected upon removal of the breathing tube), assessments to determine brain death, the set-up and management of ventilators (life-support systems), tracheal suction, and the administration of various pulmonary medications and so much more.

Performing these procedures requires close collaboration with all healthcare professionals involved in a case: physicians, nurses, case managers, lab technicians, hospice personnel, etc. Our interactions are like well-orchestrated dances that are performed on behalf of our patients to keep them alive.

As a respiratory therapist, I often spend the greater part of my twelve-hour shift managing ventilators. This is a responsibility that brings me into close and constant contact with patients and their significant others. To maximize my success, I try to establish a rapport with my patients and their family members. This becomes even more important when trying to wean the patient off life support, since they are usually awake. Family and friends are often present throughout the day and, depending on the institution, throughout the night. Thus, my interactions were not limited to the care of my patients but also their family members and significant others. Typically, a great deal of communication occurs regarding the condition of the patient and the procedures being performed on their loved one.

The array of equipment and monitors in an intensive care room is intimidating for the patient and family. This is especially true when it comes to cardiac monitors and life-support equipment. When a patient is taken off sedation, they often become keenly aware of their surroundings, including the equipment to which they are attached. Others seem to be less aware of their environment. Family and friends look at the monitors and the equipment and their ever-changing displays. Worry creeps in when alarms go off, and the numbers change. Those present in the room are very much aware of the fluctuating heart and respiratory rates, the increasing and decreasing oxygen levels, the patient's restlessness. Their grimacing, coughing, or apparent inability to interact with their loved ones is evident and disturbing. Families and patients often receive nebulous information that, at times, conflicts from different physicians and staff members.

Consequently, I feel that part of my responsibility is to teach the patient, family, and significant others. In many cases, however, the patient is extremely ill, or they are dying. Thus, the situation in which the patient, family, and friends may find themselves is one of tremendous physical, mental, emotional, and spiritual stress. It is a time of uncertainties, hope, sorrow, doubt, grief, sadness, anger, confusion, hopelessness, as well as physical, mental, and emotional exhaustion.

Facing death or the dying process of a loved one is always traumatic. It is during this chaotic and frightening time that the family is often called upon to make crucial decisions regarding their own life or that of a loved one. These decisions are often based on conflicting, confusing, and imprecise explanations regarding the case.

During my many years of practice, I have witnessed miraculous recoveries and a great deal of prolonged suffering that could have been avoided or at least lessened to some degree. What is sad is that those patients were at the end of their lives, and no amount of medical intervention could have prevented their deaths!

Death Cannot Be Denied

You and I will face anxieties concerning our end-of-life wishes. I know it is a hard subject to talk about and one that most people avoid for fear of making the inevitable occur prematurely. This is, in many ways, a taboo subject in our society regardless of age.

It is no surprise that "…when death gestures at us, we are threatened" for death threatens "…man's ontic self, that is, his existence as a being" (W. C. Tremmel 1976). In fact, there seems to be a superstitious atmosphere surrounding this topic as if talking about it would make it happen! You need to converse about these issues and make plans for the inevitable.

Death and dying are often viewed as something that will happen far in the future or to someone else, or we simply choose not to think about it. It seems that only the old die or think about the end of life. But you know that death is inevitable at any age, and to continue to avoid this topic is irresponsible. Some of you will think that discussing death is morbid. It becomes morbid only when you become fixated or obsessed with the idea of death.

We will all die. Some will die at birth, some as teens, some in the prime of life, and some struck down by devastating illnesses, infections, congenital disorders, cancers, violence, or accidents. When death approaches, whether slowly or suddenly, many of you will be caught off-guard. You will have little or no notion of what to do in such a situation. This is especially true with the younger generation.

This book is about end-of-life issues, and its sole purpose is to encourage you to think and plan so you can truly live! As I share my personal and professional experiences, I will deliberate the issues surrounding the end of life from a clinical and practical perspective.

Much has been written on these matters, but separately, and usually within academic circles. While you may find some of the subject matter to be controversial and difficult to talk about, avoiding such discussions will not make it less real. Actually, you may encounter a more painful and prolonged death for a loved one or yourself, and greater suffering for all involved if it isn't discussed soon enough. When families are thrust into such heartbreaking experiences, the scenarios generally share certain aspects: confusion, indecisiveness, anguish, pain, loneliness, and despair experienced by the critically ill, significant other, family, and friends.

Other patients have faced situations that would put Hollywood horror movies to shame. I will also share some of those stories with you. These scenarios are played-out throughout many of the scientifically advanced societies, especially here in the United States. Our society has grown technologically in leaps and bounds over the past one hundred years. The question is, have we also grown mentally, emotionally, and spiritually to the degree that would allow us to utilize our advancing technology wisely? Those that implement the many developments will say yes. They will argue that their many years of study and practice permits them to utilize the technology in a wise fashion. Over four decades of practice and observations tells me that this is not always the case.

Could it be that the healthcare professional is projecting his or her fears and uncertainties onto the patient? Is it a matter of pride, ego, the inability to admit defeat in the face of death, or the reluctance to relinquish power? Undoubtedly, the power to heal and to delay death can be a powerful aphrodisiac and an intoxicating elixir that could easily cloud one's judgment. It does feel good when you know that you have indeed saved a person's life. But we must temper that elation with the fact that we are not the overlords of life and death and that death is not a disease but a very natural process that all living things undergo.

We have indeed conquered many diseases and illnesses that once killed tens of thousands. However, we have also given birth to the myth of eternal youth and narcissistic culture of beauty and personal power; most importantly, we are made to feel as though we should live forever.

Genuinely good people in health care are caught in this technological maelstrom. We try to be as honest as possible without overstepping professional boundaries or vaguely suggested calls for silence, which are never overtly stated, nor are they written down in some policy and procedure manual. We operate based on the demands of family members and physicians. And yes, incredible recoveries and cures occur because of medical intervention, many of which I have seen throughout the course of my career.

Nonetheless, the one thing that remains unchanged is that we will all die! We may play games and try to cheat death out of its prize, but sooner or later, death will pay every one of us a visit.

I am not a morbid individual, nor am I fascinated with death and dying. It is quite the opposite. I have a tremendous zest for life! I still look upon the world with wonderment, through the eyes of a child. What I am trying to share with everyone is that we do not truly begin to live until we accept our mortality. We spend an enormous amount of energy living in the past or worrying about the future. Yet, both the past and the future are the results of what we do and what we experience each moment of our lives. Our mortality is an integral part of our existence. So, we must accept its reality. When we do, we make each day count.

The purpose of this book is to get you to think, to examine, and to plan for such an event. And, when you are done, for you to start living your life in the moment. *Planning will free you and your family of having to make incredibly important decisions at the worst possible time*. The information provided will give you a greater understanding of the medical issues that you will likely confront. Trust me when I tell you that it is not like what you see in the movies or television shows.

There are two basic issues that you will encounter when confronted with your mortality or that of someone you love. One will be the question of being resuscitated should something happen. Most people are familiar with CPR (cardiopulmonary resuscitation requires externally pumping the heart to circulate blood and manually breathing for you). CPR entails much more, as you will learn in chapter two. The second question that you will most likely encounter is that of life support (keeping you or someone you love alive with the aid of machines, a multitude of drugs, and endless procedures). I will deliberate on the pros and cons of resuscitation and other medically advanced procedures.

Please keep in mind that I am not trying to discourage you from seeking and accepting medical care and employing extreme measures such as resuscitation and other measures designed to extend your life. *These measures represent a series of medical interventions that, when applied correctly, are truly remarkable.* However, there are many situations in which life-sustaining procedures are not appropriate. These very same life-saving measures, when inappropriately applied, prolong the dying process.

There are also gray areas that have been created by modern science and technology that makes it difficult for you to come to grips with death and dying. I know, for I can write this book thanks to such measures. However, these very same life-saving procedures are often wrongfully applied for various reasons, which I will present to you later in this book. The goal is to provide you with enough actual information so you can make informed decisions for yourself or a loved one.

You will hear convincing arguments from the medical establishment for or against advanced end-of-life measures, such as CPR. *In the end, the decision is yours, and yours alone!* Please think carefully and have a heart-to-heart with your significant others regarding your wishes concerning end-of-life issues. I implore you to be inquisitive and to leave no stone unturned.

Physicians are *not* gods, nor do they have the right to deny you or your loved one of your final wishes. It is your right to question and to decide, regardless of what you may have heard. You should learn as much as possible about the health problems being faced, pre-existing chronic illnesses, prognosis, and the possible treatments, including their positive and negative effects. All decisions that you make regarding end-of-life issues can be modified or changed at any time.

Hopefully, this book will provide you with perceptual shifts that will help you see and think clearly when making these important decisions. This will give you and your family peace of mind and will allow you to live fully in the here-and-now!

⋘ ⋙

To be or not to be - that is the question:
Whether 'tis nobler in the mind to suffer
The slings and arrows of outrageous fortune,
Or to take arms against a sea of troubles,
And, by opposing, end them. To die, to sleep-
No more-and by a sleep to say we end
The heartache and the thousand natural shocks
That flesh is heir to-'tis a consummation
Devoutly to be wished.

William Shakespeare - Hamlet, Act 3 Scene 1

CHAPTER TWO

To Live or Not to Live, That is the Question

Hamlet's soliloquy eloquently and poetically describes the most basic end-of-life issue that we will all encounter, that is, to live or not to live. Although Hamlet was contemplating suicide (an act to which I am vehemently opposed), it still applies since he was thinking about whether to continue living or not. *The slings and arrows of outrageous fortune* and *The heartache and the thousand natural shocks that flesh is heir to...* could be interpreted as the suffering that a terminal illness or devastating accident could visit upon our lives at any given time. *To take up arms against a sea of troubles, and by opposing, end them* could refer to end-of-life decisions such as refusing heroic measures. As human beings, we are self-aware, and this self-awareness brings us face-to-face with "the horrendous, nonmanipulable aspects of human existence, the sense of finitude—which is to say, the human condition" (W. C. Tremmel 1976).

We are all keenly aware of our physical life with its frailties and limited timespan. Most of us, however, have become quite adept at pushing such thoughts aside as if, in doing so, it becomes less real. Yet, death and dying are part of the natural order.

We begin the journey, albeit usually a long one, when we take our first breath. The reality of our mortality spurs us to reproduce and to create and, in so doing, we leave a legacy for those that are left behind. Death, in many ways, is a driving force to live in the here-and-now. To be cognizant of our mortality is neither morbid nor fatalistic; it is a fact of life.

In the nineteenth century, Émile Durkheim proposed the theory of the collective consciousness regarding the habits, customs, and beliefs that resulted from "…social forces that are external to the individuals" (Cole 2015). Thus, death and dying are part of the collective consciousness of humanity, for it is one of those external forces that has impacted the very fabric of society. Death and dying are present at the subconscious (more so today) and conscious levels. It is an inescapable reality, and the reminders are all around us, although they usually remain in the background. And yet, all you have to do is read a book, go to the movies, turn on the television or the radio or pay attention to the world around you. We are bombarded with death and dying. It almost seems as if death and dying have been relegated to the realm of the subliminal, that is, below the level of consciousness while continuing to affect us in various ways. It seems as if we have become inured to our impermanence (at least in technologically advanced Western societies) and, in so doing, we dismiss the idea of its universality.

Death is as natural as being born and gives rise to new life. The first step on the road to a full life is to accept your mortality. In simple philosophical terms, this is an existential issue. It is one associated with your existence and the fact that you are responsible for your own life and the decisions that you make. We are quite adept at avoiding certain issues, especially those that impact us directly. I would venture to say that current trends in our society fuel this propensity toward avoidance and accepting responsibility for our decisions. Rather than accept responsibility, face reality, and resolve interpersonal and intrapersonal emotions and conflicts, we turn a blind eye or resort to other means of numbing our awareness.

Health Care Advance Directives and Durable Power of Attorney

When you face the reality of death and dying (or visit the emergency department, or upon admission, regardless of condition), you will be asked to make certain decisions on your behalf or that of a loved one. Florida law requires that healthcare providers such as hospitals, subacute nursing facilities (SNFs), long-term acute care facilities

(LTACs), home health agencies, hospices, and health maintenance organizations (HMOs) provide you with written information on health care advance directives. (*Please remember that differences exist from state to state. Therefore, I strongly recommend that you research the specific statutes pertaining to the state in which you reside.*)

According to the Florida Health Finder website (FloridaHealthFinder.gov n.d.), there are three types of advance directives: Living Will, Health Care Surrogate Designation, and Anatomical Donation. One of the first things that you will be asked is if you have a living will. A living will is legally binding while you are still alive. It is extremely valuable if you are unable to make end-of-life decisions due to an inability to communicate. It is a legal document which details your decisions regarding the care that you receive at the end of life. *Please note that a living will is not to be confused with a Last Will and Testament, which is legally binding upon your death.* The living will must be notarized and witnessed for it to be legally binding (*check your state's requirements*), and it can be revoked or modified at any time.

However, living wills can and have been challenged by family members. *So, the best way to protect your wishes is to have the document prepared through legal services and not just a notary public.* You can be as explicit as you want, and I highly recommend that you include all the things that you would want to have done to you, or not, at the end of your life.

Make sure that you include such things as DNR orders (do not resuscitate which often requires a separate document), DNI (do not intubate), whether you want other advanced procedures taken on your behalf, such as life support (both chemical and mechanical), feeding tubes, dialysis, chemotherapy, radiation therapy, surgery, etc. and anything else that comes to mind. *Please note that a DNR will not prevent you or a loved one from being intubated. Intubation can be used as a treatment of sorts due to some acute problems.*

A Health Care Surrogate Designation is a legal document that names another individual and gives them the power to make healthcare decisions if you become incapacitated. This document can also include, if you wish, instructions similar to that of the living will. You can also appoint an alternate surrogate if the first one is unable to fulfill their duty.

The third advance directive is an anatomical donation. This document defines your wishes to donate all or part of your body upon your death. These donations can take many forms, such as organs and tissue donors, or you can donate your body to science for the training of future healthcare professionals.

I strongly urge you to consider having a *Durable Power of Attorney* (DPOA) assigned legally. A DPOA remains effective even if you become incapacitated and unable to make your own decisions. This document must make it clear that it is indeed *durable*. The DPOA entitles the holder to make all decisions regarding real property, personal property, intangible property, business properties, as well as benefits and income (Online Sunshine - Official Internet Site of the Florida Legislature 2016). Please note that as of October 1, 2011, the state of Florida changed the laws regarding DPOAs. For instance, the principal (you) does not need to be incapacitated for the agent named in the document to exercise his or her powers. You can also name backup agents without needing to create other DPOAs. Unless otherwise stated, co-agents may act alone without the consent or knowledge of the other.

Finally, photocopies and electronic copies are considered valid. Think carefully before handing out copies of your DPOA. I strongly advise you not to use generic forms that are found online or in office supply stores. I have witnessed DPOAs buckle under pressure and not follow the wishes of the dying person. This has occurred due to demands from family members and the medical establishment. Choose a person as your DPOA that is trustworthy and will handle your estate and your healthcare decisions honorably.

Have your attorney create a HIPAA (Health Insurance Portability and Accountability Act of 1996) document so that your healthcare proxy can have access to your medical records. Permission to access your medical records should also appear in your DPOA document and all other healthcare-related documents.

Keep in mind the following important details regarding a do not resuscitate order:

1. A DNR order does NOT mean that you will be denied medical care, including all life-support measures.

2. You can cancel the DNR order at any time.

3. A DNR order means that, should your heart stop or should you stop breathing, no attempt will be made to resuscitate you.

4. Include some statement or clause that addresses your perception of what is acceptable or not acceptable regarding the conditions that would affect your life.

Plan and consider what you would do for yourself or a loved one when facing a catastrophic illness, disease, or a condition caused by an accident that becomes terminal. Also, consider a state in which there is no chance of recovering your previous level of functioning, resulting in your ultimate, prolonged deterioration, and demise.

I would recommend that you think in terms of quality of life. Think carefully and analyze this issue in depth, in terms of self, as well as others! You can be *alive* but trapped within a debilitating body that will no longer sustain any level of activity, or you can be *alive* and trapped in such a way that you cannot communicate with the world around you. In such cases, you will be asked to make decisions regarding medical processes and interventions that are often called heroic measures.

The term *heroic measures* refers to medical procedures aimed at either saving your life or prolonging your life and, yes, there is a difference. For example, if you are a healthy individual and you suffer an accident, an acute condition such as a heart attack or any other illness that can be treated successfully, then, by all means, fight for your life; such was the case with me. Heroic measures, in this instance, refers to saving your life. It is understandable to opt for heroic measures as long as there is some possibility of recuperation. But a sudden illness could easily turn into an end-of-life issue.

On the other hand, comorbidity factors are simultaneously occurring health problems such as kidney failure or insufficiency, advanced dementia, debilitating cardiac disease, severe hypertension, diabetes, morbid obesity, hyperlipidemia (abnormally high concentrations of fats in the blood), previous strokes, chronic liver disease such as cirrhosis, cancer with or without metastasis (the spread and formation of secondary tumors throughout the body) or end-stage chronic obstructive pulmonary disease (COPD) to name a few. Procedures designed to extend life that are performed on patients with comorbidity factors would mean prolonging life with no change in the outcome. In other words, you are prolonging your death.

Situations will vary from case to case, so question your physicians, and demand the clinical truth without personal biases. There is no prescribed format for asking this question. You must let the physicians know that you want the truth unfiltered. You need and deserve a clearly stated and truthful prognosis. Keep in mind that a projection of health status is not written in stone. It is a professional prediction of an expected outcome, and, as such, it can change over time.

Prognosis is usually fairly accurate. Death is inevitable, but its arrival and manifestation depend on a multitude of factors beyond anyone's control. Let the physician and other medical staff know that you truly understand the concept of a prognosis.

Two crucial components fall under the heading of heroic measures. One of them is CPR, and the other one is *life support*. Life support can include but is not limited to CPR, mechanical ventilation (a machine that breathes for you), feeding tubes, antibiotics, and a myriad of other chemicals, defibrillators, dialysis, all of which are designed to maintain life after the failure of one or more of your organ systems. Because of their importance, I will provide you with basic information so that you can make informed decisions regarding end-of-life issues. So, let us start with the most basic, which is CPR.

Cardiopulmonary Resuscitation—CPR Hollywood

The Hollywood version of CPR is all too common and, thus, the public's idea of CPR is largely derived from various popular television shows and movies. In the fictional constructs created for television and cinema, CPR generally occurs in a very tidy environment with a few people around, usually the heroic doctor, nurse, or paramedics and a few nondescript individuals.

There is a little commotion and drama, such as the heart monitor suddenly going flat-line and the alarm sounding. Someone yells *Code Blue* or *Call a Code*, and immediately two or three people are there. The patient's chest is pumped a few times then the paddles come out (although these are not as common as they used to be) even though their clothes are still on the person (in many shows).

The doctor or nurse calls *all clear*, and the patient is shocked. This may happen once or twice, at which point a heartbeat, as evidenced by the heart monitor that once again springs into life, is re-established, or the patient dies. The patient is rarely intubated, there is a distinct lack of controlled chaos, and the whole thing is over in record time! In a great many cases, these stories end with "…and they lived happily ever after."

These shows indicate and would have you believe, that approximately 75% of patients resuscitated live long enough to leave the hospital in good health (Span 2012) (M. Stix 2013). This portrayal is far from truth and reality! Current studies indicate that people still think that 75 percent of all CPR is successful and that 70 percent of those studied "…regularly watched medical dramas. Of these participants, 12 percent said these shows served as a reliable source of health information" (Knowles 2018).

Cardiopulmonary Resuscitation—CPR Reality

The CPR procedure performed on you or a loved one is not without risk. You should know the truth so you can make an informed decision.

CPR is administered when a person's heart has stopped functioning adequately enough to sustain life, or the person has stopped breathing, or both.

During a resuscitation attempt, you have a physician, several nurses, at least two respiratory therapists in charge of ventilation, blood gases, intubation (depending on the institution), and life-support systems, electrocardiogram technicians, laboratory personnel, and security.

At its most basic level, CPR involves manually compressing the chest to pump blood throughout the body. The procedure requires that the sternum (the flat bone located on the front part of your chest to which the ribs are attached) be compressed at least 2 inches (not less than 1.5 inches and not greater than 2.4 inches) at a rate of 100 to 120 times per minute. These compressions must be done properly to pump blood and medications to your vital organs successfully. However, these potentially life-saving compressions come with some very serious risks as you will learn later in this chapter.

CPR usually involves breathing for the person using the mouth to mouth breathing, or an Ambu Bag (a mask that goes over the nose and mouth creating a partial seal and squeezing the bag to pump oxygen into the lungs).

There is an average period of approximately six minutes before irreversible brain damage starts to occur due to *anoxia* (lack of oxygen).

The most common arrhythmias that require CPR are ventricular fibrillation, pulseless ventricular tachycardia, pulseless electrical activity, asystole, and pulseless bradycardia. The common denominator is that of little to no perfusion (blood flow). As a result, the organ systems of the body are starved of oxygen.

CPR also involves a host of medications designed to stimulate the heart into beating again and correcting an arrhythmia (abnormal electrical impulses that are fatal if not corrected). Oftentimes, CPR is performed more than once. The heart may be restarted for a while, but then it may go into some other arrhythmia that is equally life-threatening. If the heart does not respond to the chemical stimulation, then an electric shock is applied depending on the arrhythmia.

The most commonly encountered basic arrhythmias to which an electric shock can be applied during CPR are ventricular fibrillation (refers to the erratic electrical impulses that cause the lower chambers of the heart to contract in a quiver-like fashion without pumping the blood), and pulseless ventricular tachycardia (the patient can be pulseless with little to no blood flow). The amount of energy used is around three thousand volts! The reason that these arrhythmias are shocked is that they can often be converted to a normal or life-sustaining rhythm.

During CPR, the patient may require intubation to secure proper air exchange in the lungs. During intubation, an endotracheal tube (a tube about 8 inches to 10 inches long) will be inserted down the throat into the trachea, and a balloon will be inflated to seal off the windpipe. This is necessary to provide oxygen to your organs, including your brain.

There are other tubes used in the resuscitation effort, and their efficiency varies depending on their design. If you are in the hospital, you will have readily available intravenous catheters that can be used to inject various chemical compounds. However, establishing an intravenous site may be quite difficult due to the lack of blood pressure. In such cases, whether in the field or the hospital, an intraosseous device may be used. This device is normally screwed into the humerus (the long bone of the upper arm) or the tibia (shin bone of the lower leg).

Blood tests are often done, including an arterial blood gas (ABG). To perform an ABG test requires that arterial blood be obtained from various sites. Frequently during CPR, the blood is drawn from the femoral artery, which is a major artery found in the groin. This is necessary because the oxygen content of the blood drops, the carbon dioxide levels increase, and the blood becomes acidic. These are three conditions that are not conducive to life if not corrected as soon as possible.

The purpose of CPR is to re-establish life-sustaining functions, such as the circulation of blood and breathing, both of which are essential to maintaining the various organ systems in working order.

However, the truth of the matter is that the effectiveness of CPR depends on multiple factors, such as the condition that led to the cardiac or respiratory arrest, the age of the person, the state of their health, and whatever comorbidity factors are involved. Comorbidity factors can significantly affect the outcome of a resuscitation attempt.

Other crucial factors are the location in which the resuscitation occurs, and the technical proficiency of the personnel involved. The results also vary depending on whether the resuscitation attempt occurred in-hospital or out-of-hospital. Many studies have been carried out over the years to determine the efficacy of CPR. The results vary since the data is often difficult to obtain. However, there seems to be some agreement as to the results of CPR in terms of survival.

How Successful is CPR?

The data regarding successful CPR attempts may appear to be somewhat dated. The truth is that current studies indicate that little has changed when it comes to CPR. I have been practicing CPR since 1973, and I can tell you that, although advances have been made over the years, the way resuscitation is performed remains the same. Perhaps some future discoveries will truly revolutionize CPR. But, until then, we must contend with the fact that success rates for out-of-hospital CPR are about 10 percent for individuals in their forties and fifties, but the success rates drop for every decade of life: 8.1% for those in their sixties, 7.1% for those in their seventies, and about 3.3% for those in their eighties (Span 2012). In order for this success rate to occur, the "…event needs to be witnessed by bystanders, or they need to be found within seconds of collapsing and going unconscious" (Leigh 2019).

When you think about success rates, you must think in terms of the final condition of the individual. There is an enormous difference between being resuscitated and eventually regaining a fruitful and productive life or being resuscitated to end up with damaged organs (including brain damage) and a debilitating existence that is irreversible. The odds of successful resuscitation are slightly better if it occurs in-hospital.

A comprehensive thirty-year study, conducted from 1960 to 1990, revealed that little has changed regarding successful resuscitation attempts. A. Patrick Schneider (Schneider 1992) stated that the rate of success had remained between 15% and 16% with "72.9 percent of the post-CPR deaths" occurring "within 72 hours…."

You should also look at the survival rates after a successful resuscitation attempt. Per this study, almost 50% died within the first twenty-four hours, and 98% of the patients had died within thirty days of being resuscitated. Also, the success rate for CPR dramatically decreases with the length of time that the resuscitation is carried out.

In other words, the longer the resuscitation effort, the lower the success rate. In fact, CPR longer than thirty minutes has a success rate of approximately 1.2% (Schneider 1992). It has been shown that "...patients with metastatic cancer, AIDS, renal failure, sepsis, or pneumonia have less than a 5 percent chance of survival to discharge. In one study of CPR in an intensive care unit, only 3 percent of ICU patients survived the procedure" (S. R. Kaufman 2005).

Current studies indicate that the survival rates after CPR have not changed significantly. Some of the latest research indicates that a study conducted in 2012 revealed "...that only about 2% of adults who collapse on the street and receive CPR recover fully. Another from 2009 showed that anywhere from 4% to 16% of patients who received bystander CPR were eventually discharged from the hospital. About 18% of seniors who receive CPR at the hospital survive to be discharged, according to a third study" (M. Stix 2013).

CPR is considered successful if the patient is discharged from the healthcare facility. As of this update, the statistics for a successful CPR attempt conducted in a hospital are around 10.8%, with only 9% surviving with an intact neurological system (SCAFoundation 2018).

I have included these statistics on the efficacy of CPR not to dissuade you from accepting CPR but to accept it judiciously, as you will see, either for yourself or for a loved one.

Complications of CPR

You must be aware of the complications that arise as a direct result of CPR attempts. A very common problem, for example, is that of broken ribs or a cracked sternum. The sound of ribs being fractured is horrific because it sounds like branches or twigs being bent and broken.

Certain conditions will greatly increase the occurrence of fractures during CPR. For example, there is a high incidence of osteoporosis among the elderly, a condition in which the bones become brittle due to hormonal changes. Osteoporosis can be so severe that a misstep or sudden twist can cause a fracture.

Also, a prolonged deficiency of calcium and vitamin D (another cause of osteoporosis) is also conducive to fractures during CPR and prolonged use of corticosteroids, such as Prednisone and Solu-Medrol, which will also affect the bones by making them more prone to fractures.

Now, imagine what compressing the sternum 2.0 inches to 2.4 inches will do! These rib fractures can and do cause damage to internal organs such as, lacerations to the liver, spleen, and a possible hemopericardium (an accumulation of blood within the membrane that surrounds the heart and a condition that in and of itself can be fatal) (Schneider 1992).

The lungs can easily collapse as a result of a puncture from a broken rib or overly aggressive pumping of oxygen into the lungs.

Damage to the vocal cords and injury to the tracheal wall, or the surface of the windpipe during the intubation procedure, could occur. If the tube is placed into the esophagus, gastric distention can ensue, and this could lead to aspiration, among other things. Aspiration refers to the introduction of gastric (stomach) material into the lungs. Gastric substances include food, bacteria, and hydrochloric acid. This can occur prior to and during the resuscitation effort.

The result of aspiration is an instant inflammation of the bronchial passages, and the introduction of gastric content, microscopic organisms, and fluid into the lungs, all of which will further impede the exchange of gases in the lungs. Should the individual survive, they will, in many cases, be battling very serious pneumonia. It will be more difficult to deliver oxygen to the body, and carbon dioxide retention will often increase, depending on the individual case.

Also, one of the more devastating possibilities is that of permanent brain damage due to a lack of oxygen (M. Stix 2013). This is called anoxia. When this occurs, the individual will no longer be able to express himself or herself. If the anoxia is prolonged, it could easily result in brain death. In this situation, life cannot be sustained without the aid of a ventilator.

We should all remember the case of Terry Schiavo. Terry collapsed due to cardiac arrest resulting from a potassium imbalance at the age of twenty-seven (Cline 2016). She was successfully resuscitated but had suffered irreversible brain damage. As a result, Terry Schiavo spent the next fifteen years in a persistent vegetative state. According to Cheryl Arenella MD, MPH (Arenella n.d.), a "vegetative state exists when a person is able to be awake but is totally unaware. A person in a vegetative state can no longer 'think,' reason, relate meaningfully with his/her environment, recognize the presence of loved ones, or 'feel' emotions or discomfort. The higher levels of the brain are no longer functional. A vegetative state is called 'persistent' if it lasts for more than four weeks."

Although much controversy exists surrounding the case of Terry Schiavo, the fact remains that upon her autopsy, it was revealed that her brain was approximately half of its normal weight. This condition severely impaired her (Grady 2005).

The severity of her brain injury due to a lack of oxygen left her with the following impairments:

- Totally dependent on others.
- Unable to eat or drink without choking or aspirating.

- Unable to speak.

- Unable to control bladder and bowel functions.

- Able to have periods of wakefulness and sleep.

- Able to sneeze, cough, cry, and smile.

- Able to automatically respond to touch, sound, and light.

The abilities exhibited by Terry Schiavo are all automatic responses that did not require thinking (Arenella n.d.). Newborn babies sneeze, cough, cry, and smile, and they also respond to touch, sound, and light. However, these are all automatic responses that do not require any thinking processes. As the newborn develops, the ability to cognitively interact with their environment comes into play. When this is lost as a result of brain injury, such as anoxia, cognitive cannot be recovered.

My heart goes out to her family. I can only imagine the anguish and pain that they experienced. Their decisions were based on love, regardless of whether we agree with them or not. Nonetheless, one crucial question remains. Would you like to see yourself or a loved one in the same condition as Terry Schiavo?

The possibility of a severely decreased quality of life exists, especially as you get older. The occurrence of those things described is such that many physicians will decline CPR. "Ken Murray argues that physicians decline these 'heroic' measures for intellectual reasons.

He argues that we know the data, which includes a study that reported that, of people who receive CPR, only 8% are successfully resuscitated. (Of that 8 %, only a portion of them return to their previous full function.)" (Yang 2013).

Physicians are not alone in this decision. Many professionals in the medical field will tell you that they do not want to be resuscitated!

Life Support and Mechanical Ventilation

Should you or a loved one survive a resuscitation attempt, the most likely scenario that would follow is that of being on life support. However, you do not have to have been resuscitated to end up on life support. Life support entails the use of different therapies or interventions designed to maintain biological life or the life of your body (note that this does not address other issues such as the mental, emotional, and spiritual aspects of your being).

Life support can take many forms depending on the individual case. The most commonly known form is that of the person on a ventilator, which is the modern version of the iron-lung. This form of life support is known as mechanical ventilation. It is a wonderful technology that aids in preserving life. It is truly a miracle worker when it comes to getting you through a rough patch such as severe pneumonia, an exacerbation of COPD (emphysema, asthma, bronchiectasis, and many others), and post-operative complications to name a few. If it weren't for the ventilator, I would not be here today. On the other hand, mechanical ventilation could, depending on the patient's condition, prolong their death!

Unfortunately, the instance of prolonging the dying process of a fellow human being is more common than you would imagine. To be on mechanical ventilation, you must have been intubated. As I mentioned in the previous section, the process of intubation carries its risks, such as damaged vocal cords, chipped teeth, and aspiration (when inserted into the esophagus instead of the windpipe).

Also, the size of the endotracheal tube varies. For example, adult endotracheal tubes normally range from 6.0mm to 10mm in diameter or 0.24 inches to 0.39 inches. In other words, you will be breathing through a fat straw. When weaning attempts are carried out, the patient's sedation is turned off, and you become aware of your surroundings (as if looking at the world through a thick fog) and whatever pains you may be experiencing.

Now you are awake, in pain, and unable to talk (the tube in your throat prevents you from talking). When the ventilator is working, the air is forced into your lungs. But, when the weaning process starts, you must do all the work, albeit with some assistance from the ventilator. So, visualize being awake, and fully aware of your surroundings, while breathing through a fat straw! Imagine the emotional upheavals that would be experienced by you (the patient) and your loved ones present. Now throw in some phlegm or lung secretions, and you can easily conjure up what you would feel.

During this time, a pulmonary lavage may be necessary. This requires the introduction of five to fifteen cubic centimeters of saline (salt solution) into the endotracheal tube with subsequent suctioning. This feels, to the patient, as if you were trying to drown him or her! The introduction of the suction catheter can cause further damage to the tracheal wall (windpipe), increase the risk of infection, and elicit an uncontrollable urge to cough.

After approximately fourteen days, physicians will start considering performing a tracheotomy (an opening that is surgically created in your throat, which includes the insertion of a tracheostomy tube). This will facilitate breathing, weaning, and, in most cases, it is a temporary condition because the tracheostomy tube can be removed, and the stoma (or hole in the trachea) will close and this will allow the patient to breathe normally. *Remember, however, that when you have entered the process of dying, being on a ventilator will not change the prospects but prolong the dying phase.*

Another issue that may be encountered is that you may develop an inability to swallow liquids or solids properly. This may result in food or liquid being introduced into the lungs, thereby causing some serious problems such as aspiration pneumonia. If you are lucky, you may be able to eat a soft-diet or pureed foods and drink thickened liquids. Or, you may be fed through a tube.

Life support is not just mechanical ventilation, but it is typically accompanied by a host of other interventions designed to keep your body alive. You and your family must choose whether to accept the use of such heroic measures. Just remember that all choices regarding life support or the use of heroic measures are optional. Besides resuscitation and mechanical ventilation, these measures can include any or all the following:

Artificial Nutrition, Hydration, Tube Feedings, Intravenous Feeding

Marianne Duda, MS, RDN, LDN, CNSC Clinical Nutritionist, wrote:

> When people cannot, will not or should not eat, the medical team considers alternative ways to keep a person hydrated and fed. When used near the end of life, these therapies are considered heroic measures by some, and by others, simply essential for life.
>
> Usually, an IV line is inserted into a vein in the back of the hand or forearm to instill hydration and medications. Depending on the person's condition, a special IV catheter may be

tunneled through the arm or inserted directly into the larger veins of the neck or chest. Nutrients, hydration, and medications can then be infused directly into the large vein (superior vena cava) that empties into the heart, then pumped throughout the body. Feeding into this large vein is known as parenteral nutrition (PN) and is used when the stomach and bowels are not able to digest and absorb essential nutrients. Other names for IV feeding include total parenteral nutrition (TPN), central parenteral nutrition (CPN), total nutrient admixture (TNA), Hyperal, Hyperalimentation, peripheral parenteral nutrition (PPN) or home parenteral nutrition (HPN).

Alternatively, a feeding tube may be inserted through the nose, mouth, or through an opening made in the abdomen to access the stomach or small intestines. Tube feeding is also known as enteral nutrition, or by the type and placement of the feeding tube. These include nasogastric (NG) orogastric (OG), nasojejunal (Dubhoff or NJ), gastrostomy (G-tube), percutaneous endoscopic gastrostomy (PEG), percutaneous endoscopic gastrojejunostomy (PEG/J), and jejunostomy (J-tube). It is not uncommon for one to receive both types of therapy. Hydration and medications are often provided through an IV, while nutrient-rich liquids (and some medications) are given through a feeding tube.

The issues surrounding these life-support measures are even more controversial since food has always been associated with life. As such, it elicits quite an array of mental, emotional, and spiritual angst, such as the fear of letting a loved one die of hunger or thirst.

> As discussed throughout this book, the most difficult decisions are made when determining if the end of life is near. Should we feed? Should we keep our loved ones hydrated? A difficult decision for family members and loved ones is not made any easier by the health-care team. Dehydration does not just occur with the inability to take fluids by mouth but also occurs with high fevers, losses through the gut (diarrhea, watery stools, ostomy output, fistulas), and through draining wounds and environmental factors. These factors can contribute to an end of life scenario, so should adequate hydration and replacement of fluid losses be withheld? Health-care professionals are taught that TPN and tube feeding should be withheld when there is a poor or terminal prognosis or where aggressive therapy is not desired, but they don't tell us 'not desired' by whom? (Duda 2017).

Marianne Duda's writing reinforces the need to be thoroughly informed both with a diagnosis, as well as a prognosis, since, in many cases, these procedures can save your life. However, in others, all it will do is prolong the dying process. It is interesting to note that research has shown that these forms of feeding do not provide comfort and that without them, patients can die comfortably (Life Support Choices 2011). Artificial feeding can quite often result in aspiration into the lungs (with the exception of the dobhoff tube), which results in complicated pneumonia. Research shows that "…dehydration in the end stage of a terminal illness is a very natural and compassionate way to die" (Dunn 2016).

Dialysis

This procedure involves the insertion of a dialysis catheter. It is inserted into the subclavian (major vein found under the collar bone), internal jugular (a major vein found on the side of your neck), or the femoral vein (major vein found in the groin area). The dialysis catheter can only be used between two to six weeks for an acute condition or a newly acquired chronic one. For a chronic condition, a much more extensive surgical procedure is required. Dialysis for the chronically ill or dying patient will only prolong the process of dying (Definition of Catheter - hemodialysis 2012). These procedures entail risks, such as internal bleeding and a pneumothorax. A pneumothorax refers to a lung collapse due to a puncture or rupture. A pneumothorax will then require another surgical intervention to insert tubes to re-expand the injured lung.

Pacemakers

These small electronic devices are surgically implanted into the chest wall to regulate slow or erratic heartbeats. There are various risks associated with this procedure: "Because pacemaker implantation is an invasive surgical procedure, internal bleeding, infection, hemorrhage, and embolism are all possible complications. Infection is more common in patients with temporary pacing systems" and "The placing of the leads and electrodes during the implantation procedure also presents certain risks for the patient. The lead or electrode could perforate the heart or cause scarring or other damage. The electrodes can also cause involuntary stimulation of nearby skeletal muscles" (Youngson 2016).

Surgical Procedures

I have already mentioned a few: tracheotomy, biopsies, insertions of various catheters (both venous and arterial), various drains, pacemaker insertion, and, depending on the individual case, major surgery.

Pharmaceuticals

This is a difficult subject to address because of the hundreds of medicines that are available. It is beyond the scope of this book to list all the chemical compounds that are used in the medical field. Suffice it to say that the powerful drugs used can and do have serious side effects that can be damaging to various organ systems of the body.

Lab and Radiology Procedures

Numerous daily blood and urine analyses, as well as a multitude of radiology tests that range from a simple x-ray, CT-Scan, or MRI to the more complex interventional procedures that are performed by an interventional radiologist.

Tubes, Tubes, and More Tubes!

This category includes, but is not limited to intravenous, arterial, rectal, urinary bladder, feeding tubes (NG or nasogastric, OG or orogastric), various surgically implanted drains, endotracheal tubes, tracheostomy tubes, and more.

Hopefully, this will give you an idea of some of the medical procedures involved in end-of-life interventions. This is just the beginning since, in making such important decisions, you must also consider the financial impact upon either yourself or your family. End-of-life measures are extremely costly, both personally and to society.

Financial Impact

My personal journey through this nightmare included the emergency department, eventual surgical procedures, and life support (including mechanical ventilation) for two weeks, four days on the medical-surgical floor, and six weeks of heavy-duty antibiotic therapy at home, costing an excess of $250,000. This did not include extraneous bills from outside agencies such as radiologists, laboratory charges, medications, follow-up visits with physicians, etc. Although we had an excellent insurance policy, it was not enough.

The total financial impact, including hospitalization, continued IV therapy for six weeks, and loss of income was probably around $50,000. Even with the insurance, my wife and I had to cash in our 401K to pay our bills, and we sold 3.5 acres of land that we had purchased for our future. We also received help from family and friends, and the apartment complex in which we were living waived one month's rent. We were fortunate but imagine those that have no insurance or an insurance policy that does not cover what ours did. This occurred over eighteen years ago and it is much more expensive today!

Not long ago, I took my wife to the emergency room because of some lower abdominal pain. She was there for approximately two hours and was discharged home. The bill was more than $17,000. I know from experience that when confronted with a devastating illness, the bill can run into the millions depending on a variety of factors.

I offer these examples to illustrate the financial impact that illness can have on your life. When the issue addressed is a critical one, the financial impact is mind-blowing. Without insurance or an excellent support structure, the financial nightmare could extend beyond imagination.

The issues surrounding the financial aspects of death and dying must be considered, especially today. Such catastrophic scenarios could easily devastate your loved ones financially. Let us take a short journey through the financial aspects of the end of life.

I cannot go into an itemized and detailed account of the costs having to do with the end of life since these will vary significantly from case to case. This may sound calloused and impersonal but believe me when I tell you that a good number of dying patients are worried about what their loved ones will be going through because of their medical condition. If you have reached the end of your life, what is the point of incurring a tremendous amount of debt if, in the end, the outcome will not change?

You should keep in mind that the costs at the end of life are not just financial, but also physical, mental, emotional, and spiritual. I will start with the financial aspects of death and dying. Let me assure you that I am not putting a price tag on life. Life is priceless as long as there is quality! However, this is a topic that must be brought to light, since you and I and everyone else in this world will come face-to-face with this reality.

The financial issues I highlight are the unnecessary costs acquired at the end of life. They address medical interventions that do not change the final expected outcome of the patient. It saddens me to see a great number of people today spend their last days in an intensive care unit surrounded by machines, constant testing, and a multitude of other indignities. Patients are subjected to a constant barrage of interventions of all sorts designed to either extend the life of their body or investigate what else is going on in their body. Much of what occurs in hospitals today is cookie-cutter medicine, which leads to unnecessary procedures and expenses and unprecedented negative outcomes.

For instance, when a patient meets the criteria for the implementation of a "Sepsis Protocol," one of the indications is to utilize a fairly large amount of intravenous fluids. There is scientific evidence to support such actions. Research shows that such interventions definitely improve mortality rates. The issue lies in such protocols being used judiciously. It should be up to the physician to implement the protocol. According to Diana J Kelm, M.D. et al. (Kelm, et al. 2015) our "…study found that persistent clinical and radiologic evidence of fluid overload was associated with an increase in the acute need for fluid-related medical interventions, hospital mortality…" and more.

This study goes on to state that the use of such protocols has been associated with an increase in medical interventions and costs resulting from various complications, increases in the need for diuretics and thoracentesis (removal of fluid with a needle) due to pleural effusions or the accumulation of fluids between the two membranes surrounding the lungs, pulmonary edema (lungs fill up with fluid) and increases in blood pressure (Kelm, et al. 2015). Such a condition could easily result in the patient having to be intubated and placed on mechanical ventilation and other life-support measures.

These added measures carry their own risks. They increase the length of stay in the hospital and incur increased charges, both of which could have been avoided. The physician should be the one making such decisions on a patient-to-patient basis.

Unfortunately, physicians are being stripped of their ability to manage their patients' illnesses as taught. Instead, the course of their work is being dictated by external policies put into effect by hospital administrations. I have taken care of patients that were critically ill and dying a very prolonged death. These patients and their families ended up with astronomical financial costs ranging from $250,000 to $1,500,000 only to prolong their deaths.

Were they billed these massive amounts? Probably not, since health insurance would have paid a portion of such bills. Did the hospital absorb some, or all, of the cost depending on whether or not the patient had some type of health insurance? The answer is, yes! Did the patients get billed for a large chunk of the money due? You bet! And what they received for their money was the privilege of dying or watching a loved one die a long and often agonizing death, one piece at a time.

We must all consider the total effect of our journey through the end of life. It is easy to say that saving one's life or that of a loved one is worth all the money in the world. This is true if the patient's condition is reversible or the illness curable.

I have had the pleasure throughout my career of being able to help many patients come off life support and resume their lives while working alongside excellent teams of nurses and physicians. Unfortunately, I have also watched that very same technology extend the process of dying and suffering. It is heart-wrenching to watch patients and their loved ones go through this process to no avail. Yet, as healthcare professionals, we are dedicated to our patients' wellbeing and continue to do the best that we can, even when we know the outcome. Keep in mind, however, that the cost of life-prolonging procedures will vary according to the medical issues being addressed.

To give you an idea from my own profession, an ABG, which is extensively used when a patient is on life support, will cost between $1,200 and $2,000 per test, and the price will vary from institution to institution. This lab test is done, in many cases, on a routine basis (at least once a day), and it is often performed several times during a twenty-hour period. This blood test is often necessary to determine how well the lungs are working and how well other compensatory systems, such as the kidneys, are functioning. Is this test used excessively and unnecessarily? Absolutely! Is the patient charged? Absolutely!

For example, to determine the acidity or alkalinity of the blood, an arterial blood gas is not necessary, since this test can be performed with venous blood, and there are other non-invasive methods of monitoring oxygen and carbon dioxide levels. There are many other instances when this test is used inappropriately. However, keep in mind that there are driving influences behind all situations. A powerful force that has adversely impacted the practice of medicine, the healthcare industry, and insurance costs is our litigious society and the unwillingness of lawmakers to change existing laws. One of the many results is that a lot of physicians are forced to order and repeat tests and/or perform procedures for fear of being sued.

So, if you are in the intensive care unit and on a ventilator for fourteen days (not unusual), the charge for arterial blood gases alone could be around $28,000 (if it is only done once per day). If you are being weaned off life support, the price tag could be as high as $42,000 over fourteen days. The ventilator charge can vary from $1,500 per day (Dasta, et al. 2005) to over $3,000 per day, depending on the hospital and the area of the country. So, the charge for ventilator support can be $21,000 or higher. Therefore, you can easily acquire a charge of $63,000 on just these two items.

Now, let's move on to room and board charges. Room and board charges for intensive care unit stays can range anywhere from $11,000 per day if you are on a ventilator or around $7,000 per day without a ventilator. After the second day, it decreases from about $5,000 to approximately $4,000 and stabilizes after the third day at about $3,500 (Dasta, et al. 2005).

These prices, as I have mentioned before, will vary from hospital to hospital, state to state, and general area of the country. Please note that in this very simplistic scenario, the medical bill at the end of your fourteen days will be over $100,000. Although some of this data will appear to be dated, current studies indicate that the expense will indeed exceed $100,000 (Michael P Donahoe 2012).

If you add radiology services (x-rays, MRIs, CT-scans, etc.), lab tests, possible surgical interventions, medications, oxygen, and an endless array of supplies (tubes of all sorts, various kits, bandages, Band-Aids, and much more) you can see why your bill could easily be over $200,000. I have seen some exceed one million dollars.

The portion of the bill you will be responsible for will depend on what your insurance pays and how aggressively the hospital and other independently contracted services will try to collect from you and your family. Your inability to pay may affect your credit ratings for years, which, in turn, can affect your ability to be employed. If the hospital or any other entity involved decide to take legal action against you, the effects are devastating.

An article published in The Fiscal Times stated that "43 percent of Medicare recipients spend more than the total value of their assets, excluding their home, on out-of-pocket medical costs. And 25 percent spend everything they have – or more than they have – including the value of their home" (Rosenberg 2012). The cost of medical care skyrockets during the last five years of life, during which time the household finances are depleted, leaving the surviving spouse with an untenable debt added to the sorrow of having lost a loved one. Amid the mental, emotional, and spiritual turmoil, families could face financial hardships.

What saddens me is this: studies show these heroic measures had "'no meaningful impact' on the outcome" (Alfonsi 2009). I know that this is NOT an easy topic to talk about, due to the mental, emotional, and spiritual variables of the individual facing the end of life, or his or her loved ones. The topic becomes truly painful if you find yourself having to consider the removal of life support.

Therefore, there is one question that you will need to ask yourself and one that you should revisit as conditions change over time: *Will you, in the end, be prolonging life or prolonging death either for yourself or someone you love?* It is up to each individual and their family to answer this most difficult question. If you arm yourself with accurate information regarding the condition and prognosis of the patient, you will avoid the uncertainty that can cloud your thinking. Know the type of disease or illness, comorbidity factors, and the person's overall health prior to the event. Remember, it is paramount to respect and act upon the person's expressed desires.

CB EO

Death—the last sleep? No, it is the final awakening.

Sir Walter Scott

CHAPTER THREE

Prolonging Death or Prolonging Life: Food for Thought

If you or a loved one are in good overall physical health, then life-support measures would be advisable. For example, at the time of this writing, I am sixty-seven, and my wife is sixty-eight. We are in excellent health, have no major comorbidity factors, and are physically and mentally active. Spiritually, we are quite aware that life does not end with physical death, so we acknowledge our mortality while embracing our lives. Should an acute health crisis occur, we would consider life-support measures. However, should an acute condition turn chronic and debilitating in such a way that we would not be able to use our minds or take care of ourselves, we would, without hesitation, terminate life support.

For you to arrive at a decision such as the one previously described, you should honestly assess your current state of existence or that of a loved one. You need to think holistically (analyze the situation from all angles) and discuss everything with your family and significant other.

The Issue of Communication

The first step for you to achieve is a clear understanding of your condition or that of someone you love. You need to be aware of the disease processes going on in the body. Next, you must request from your physicians clear and unbiased statements of the ongoing health issues. Make it clear to them that you want the truth, not some sugar-coated version of what they think you will be able to handle. However, *you must be prepared to hear the truth.* Do not be angry with the physician that is honest and forthcoming with the facts. Not wanting to hear the truth is like burying your head in the sand, but the reality is still there waiting for you. Not knowing the veracity of the case does not change the outcome.

Let me reiterate the fact that physicians are regular people like you and me that happen to have studied medicine. They are not infallible. The vast majority of doctors have your best interest at heart, but they are just as human as you and me. Because of this, most doctors have personal biases, pride, egocentric personalities, religious or non-religious beliefs, etc. All of which will usually remain undisclosed and for very good reasons.

All healthcare personnel practice some degree of distancing from the cases for which we are responsible. It is acceptable because it establishes a sense of trust between you and your physician, as well as other healthcare personnel. To others, it may appear as if we are distant or even cold. The truth, however, is that allowing our feelings, thoughts, and emotions to surface would only cloud our judgment. This is designed to reassure you and instill some degree of confidence. You would feel rather uneasy if you become aware of your physician's emotional state or of what they thought of the world.

However, due to time constraints and, in many cases, poor communication skills with the patients and family, the quality and quantity of information are often inadequate. I have been present in hundreds of such encounters and have been witness to their discomfort and unease when approaching such topics as death and dying. The most common feedback that I receive from patients is that of a lack of communication, especially from the physicians.

The responsibility of establishing a good exchange of information also falls on the shoulders of the patients and the family. Many patients and family members have *selective hearing*, since they tend to focus on aspects of a conversation that sound hopeful. Listen to the doctor carefully and ask questions. Better yet, write down the questions you want to be answered. Do not accept anything other than a truthful and complete answer to your questions.

For example, during my hospitalization in 2001, I was fortunate to have had an amazing primary physician, two excellent pulmonologists, nurses, and respiratory therapists. My wife was at my side every day throughout most of the day and night. Regardless of her presence, the transmission of information from the pulmonologists was lacking, and it almost seemed as if they were avoiding her. My wife, who is 5'1", managed to corral one of the pulmonologists and demanded that she be kept informed. He was quite optimistic about my eventual recovery, and after that encounter, he kept my wife informed.

About one week after being placed on a ventilator, the other pulmonologist informed my wife that she ought to gather the family together since I was gravely ill and that I might not make it. My wife got angry and banned him from seeing me. While he is an excellent pulmonologist and was correct in his assessment (since my illness carried a mortality rate between 40% to 50%), her issue was with his casual announcement and the conflicting viewpoints between the physicians. The lack of depth of the information given, the avoidance of the family (in this case, my wife), and the way it was delivered made an already very stressful situation worse.

Doctors do disagree, and this is to be expected from time to time. If your physician is part of a group, you may see another doctor if yours is unavailable. However, he or she should defer to your primary physician, and the physicians should discuss differences of opinion or approach privately. Their communication should avoid giving the patient and family conflicting messages, such as what occurred in my case. All medical personnel and hospital administrations should keep in mind that most people have a built-in lie detector. They can sense when a healthcare practitioner is being insincere or is not forthcoming with information.

Many hospitals love to sell and implement scripted responses to various situations that may arise with the patient and family members. I can tell you from personal experience that it does not work since many patients have made it known to me. Lying to the patient and their family, whether completely or partially, is misleading, disrespectful, patronizing, condescending, extremely poor public relations, and can lead to litigation since all that has been accomplished is angering people!

It is wrong for a physician to feel that all of their patients and family members are incapable of understanding medical issues or disease processes. This may have been the mentality over forty years ago, but not today. The truth is that medical information is readily available, and people research issues surrounding a particular illness, medications and their interactions, recovery periods, and possible outcome.

Patients and their families may not possess the depth of medical knowledge of a physician, nurse, or therapist, but they may have a better grasp of the situation than they are given credit. I have seen many physicians react with anger and resentment when questioned by the patient or a family member. This is unprofessional and relies on an outdated mindset. Besides, it is your right to question the validity of all things being done to you or to someone you love.

Some physicians may have a difficult time dealing with death and dying, for they are taught to save lives and to heal. This is in part because medical schools give little training to physicians regarding end-of-life issues, and, to make matters worse, we live in a society that is inclined to negate or obscure the reality of death (Balaban 2000). Research reveals that physicians "typically receive little guidance on how to communicate with dying patients and their families" (Balaban 2000). Dr. Atul Gawande mentions that the issues surrounding our finitude were not included in the curriculum. He goes on to say that our "…textbooks had almost nothing on aging or frailty or dying, how the process unfolds, how people experience the end of their lives and how it affects those around them" (A. Gawande 2014). Also, "…there is still little discussion in medical school of the effects of medical technology on people's lives" (J. a. Fitzpatrick 2010).

A considerable number of doctors avoid interacting with family members as much as possible, especially when the outcome is not good. Thus, many physicians find it exceedingly difficult to accept death, and the way your health issues are addressed will be colored or biased based on their personalities, training, experience, and belief system. This issue involves not just doctors but other medical personnel as well.

The death of a patient is an event for which we are all ill-prepared to handle at various levels. Professionally, doctors, nurses, and respiratory therapists do not possess the adequate training required to meet the mental, emotional, and spiritual needs of their patients. Our biomedical educational system provides a wide array of technical training designed to treat and cure what ails the physical body while other training modalities are focused on prolonging life. It is a "…feature of modern medicine that 'we always want to fix, fix, fix,'" and that death is viewed "…as the ultimate failure" (Jason 2018).

I must congratulate the Boston College, Connell School of Nursing, for instituting the "…the semester-long End of Life Simulation Program" (Goldthrite 2016). This powerful simulation puts the students face-to-face with death and dying and helps to soften the impact (as much as possible) of continued exposure to such stressful situations. I only wish that such programs became the norm rather than the exception. The field is not devoid of course material dealing with this subject. There are excellent modules available that address such issues as hospice care, palliative care, advanced directives, documentation, caring for patients at the end of life, and secondary traumatic stress. Most schools include the work of Elizabeth Kübler-Ross and the five stages of grief. However, the majority of these classes are based on classroom lectures and do not provide personal exposure, which would allow the student to

"...address their own feelings about death and dying" (Goldthrite 2016). This is unfortunate since doctors, nurses, and respiratory therapists will have to confront the death of their patients.

One nursing student that was interviewed mentioned the fact that we "...never really talk about what it feels like to go through the grieving process from the viewpoint of the healthcare provider..." (Heilweil 2016).

I will never forget what it felt like trying to resuscitate my first ventilator patient and their subsequent death. I performed my duties as expected, and, in the end, I quickly withdrew to an empty room with tears in my eyes. I have also comforted fellow therapists and nurses that were distressed after having dealt with the death of their patients. Intellectually we may be prepared to handle such situations, but nothing really prepares you for the mental, emotional, and spiritual impact that occurs when facing death and dying.

Throughout my career as a respiratory therapist, I do not recall any discussions after going through the aforementioned scenarios. How can we properly address the needs of the dying patient and the patient's family when we are having difficulties ourselves?

Respiratory therapists are usually involved with the vast majority of dying patients in a variety of ways. They form an integral part of the multidisciplinary team providing clinical assessments, forming part of the rapid response team, CPR, and various facets of life support such as intubation, ventilatory support, performing various tests, brain-death determinations, and terminal extubations. As a result, they are in close contact with the dying patient as well as the patient's family. And yet, respiratory therapists are often left out when it comes to discussing the issues related to the decision to stop life support.

Like doctors and nurses, they are taught to analyze a situation and then proceed to fix it, but no training is given as to what to do when a patient reaches that point when nothing more can be done (Chandler 2019). In most institutions, it is the responsibility of the respiratory therapist to withdraw life-support ventilation, and these terminal weans take their toll at the mental, emotional, and spiritual levels.

When I was first asked to terminate life support on one of my patients, I refused. I had a difficult time coming to terms with terminating life support because my job was to assist and prolong life. Over time, this can lead to "…burnout, stress, and increased turnover" (Mahan 2019). These conditions can easily lead to what is called "compassion fatigue." It is a condition resulting from the empathy, and related stressors felt for the suffering of others in your care, especially with patients at the end of life.

In other words, professionals "…regularly exposed to the traumatic experiences of the people they service, such as health care, emergency and community service workers, are particularly susceptible to developing…"

(Joss 2016) compassion fatigue. I was fortunate in that I was better equipped to handle death and dying because of my diverse background, which included complementary healing modalities that dealt with the spiritual aspects of this topic. As a result, I was often asked to speak with family members regarding the various choices surrounding a terminal patient.

Others, however, were not involved, and they shied away from such interactions because they felt inadequate, through no fault of their own, to address such sensitive issues. And yet, they were still vulnerable to the repeated exposure to not only the suffering of their patients but to facing their patient's final moments.

Regardless of such continued exposure, one study showed that 93.8% "…participated in a terminal extubation…" and that few would actually "…speak directly with the patient and/or family about end-of-life care (10.8%) or are comfortable with end-of-life discussions with the patient and/or family (29.2%)" (Strickland 2016). Physicians and nurses are aware of the important role that respiratory therapists play when it comes to handling patients at the end of life. Unfortunately, most therapists (and I have witnessed this) feel left out and under-appreciated (Brown-Saltzman 2010).

This lack of training and exposure to the processes associated with death and dying can adversely impact the communication that must occur between the medical personnel, the patient, and the family. This situation leads to misunderstandings, anger, resentment, confusion, poor decisions on the part of the patient and family, and, in some cases, litigation. The following anecdote illustrates this issue:

I took care of a ninety-seven-year-old patient that had entered the stage of actively dying. The patient was unresponsive, blood pressure was low, as was the heart rate. Family members had made the patient a DNR, and they had all come to terms with their loved one's dying and had said their goodbyes. Hospice had been called in for an assessment. Throughout the day, one physician came in and talked the family out of hospice services and told them that he did not think that it was her time to die. Next, another physician came in and ordered that the patient be placed on Bipap, which is a form of non-invasive ventilation. This physician stated that just because she was old, it did not mean that she was dying. The Bipap treatment reversed the accumulation of carbon dioxide and increased oxygenation. Carbon dioxide has a narcotic-like effect in high concentrations, which is something that happens naturally when an individual is dying. Several days later, the patient was taken off the Bipap and placed on an oxygen mask. Her skin had suffered some breakdown as a result of the pressure exerted by the mask.

In the end, the patient's level of response remained minimal. She would briefly open her eyes and close them again, and there were little to no purposeful movements. Her respirations continued to be labored as they were before the heroic interventions. Thankfully, she remained a DNR, and all that was accomplished was prolonging her death, a natural process that commenced about a week earlier.

Days later, after seeing no improvements, the family asked for hospice once more. Hospice came in and assessed the patient. She was to go home the following day, but she passed away the night before. I knew that she was getting ready to move on because I saw her open her eyes and look at her devoted family (something she had not done for a long time). She knew that her family had finally accepted the inevitable (she was not unconscious) and that they were at peace.

I truly believe that most doctors are honest human beings who are sincerely interested in your wellbeing. I do not for one moment believe that these physicians had anything other than the patient's best interest at heart. I know these physicians well, and I know that they truly care for their patients. However, I also believe that their judgment was clouded due to their own personal viewpoints.

One physician did not *feel* that the patient was dying, and the other physician had *forgotten* that old age leads to the end of life. If you live to your nineties or beyond, you are living, as they say, on borrowed time. Old age entails the deterioration of organ systems and the inability of the body to repair itself. Thus, you can be in relatively good health, but a specific illness could propel you to the point of no return. What occurs is that the body is unable to cope with the onslaught of a serious illness, and a rapid decline ensues that often ends in a debilitated state that eventually triggers the dying process.

Another issue to remember is that a physician's success in his or her practice often involves referrals from other physicians. Consequently, some may worry about referrals and may, therefore, perform procedures because they were asked by another physician and not necessarily because they feel it is necessary.

Are these common practices? No, they are not! Most physicians are honest and conscientious individuals that will do what they feel is in your best interest. I know physicians that have rejected procedures that they did not believe would benefit the patient. *You, on the other hand, must think about what is in your best interest or that of someone you love.* Remember that it is up to you and you alone to decide.

It is, therefore, imperative for you to have a clear understanding of what is going on and why. Be informed as to why certain procedures or treatments are required and understand why certain medications are being prescribed. Research the subject matter independently or have someone you trust do it for you. You do need, however, a realistic forecast based on your diagnosis. You must be firm when asking for clear, unbiased, and concise assessments from all physicians involved in the case. If they are bothered by your requests, then it is time for you to discuss the issues with them or get another physician that is willing to honor your wishes. It is perfectly acceptable for you to get a second or third opinion. Make sure that you talk to the nurses, respiratory therapists, case managers, and social workers. As you obtain the information necessary for you to make an informed decision, carefully consider the outcome in terms of quality of life instead of merely being alive.

Quality of Life

Living a meaningful life and *being alive* are two different things. You can be braindead or in a persistent vegetative state, and you would be alive. Or, you could be bedridden, unable to talk or perform the simplest of tasks, but you are alive. Think carefully about what you value about your life and what it means to you or a loved one.

As a family member dealing with the dying of a loved one, I recommend that you exercise empathy. Put yourself in their place and the suffering that they are undergoing without any meaningful change in outcome. Remember, the question of whether life is worth living or not is a question that is not asked in medicine (S. R. Kaufman 2005).

Based on personal experience throughout my career, the question of quality of life rarely comes up in end-of-life discussions. This makes it important that you express to your family what you do or do not want to be done to you or a loved one. You should also address these things with your doctors. Let the nurses and therapists know your wishes. It will ensure that your desires are expressed and conveyed promptly. Once you have made your decision, you must make sure that your doctors honor your wishes.

How We Prolong the Dying Process

I cared for a patient who was on life support, including mechanical ventilation, and the entire gamut that goes along with it. The patient had a long history of alcoholism and had many comorbidity factors. We were unable to wean this patient from the ventilator. The patient's sister, a medical professional, wanted to remove him from the ventilator, and one of the physicians on the case refused. The issue, in this case, was not the refusal but the reasoning behind it. The doctor refused based on the belief that the sister did not have her brother's best interest at heart, a mere supposition since no evidence existed. This attitude and behavior is patronizing and condescending at best.

In this case, the physician allowed personal feelings to prevail and cloud his judgment in the decision-making process. The worst part is that the doctor was accusing the sister, directly or indirectly, of wanting to end the burden of caring for her alcoholic sibling, without knowing anything about her. His behavior is a testament to the fact that physicians are human. Naturally, the physician's opinions were not voiced to the sister of the patient, but the statement was made to some of the medical personnel that happened to be present, including me.

As you may know, fear of retribution is a powerful incentive to maintain silence. Nonetheless, medical professionals try, in many subtle ways, to help the patient and family by discussing end-of-life options such as DNR, DNI, comfort measures, and hospice. We also approach the subject indirectly in an effort to open a dialogue and talk to the family and/or the patient. As we remain observant, we look for clues that tell us that it is time to address end-of-life issues gently.

A few years ago, I witnessed an extreme and rare example of a patient's legal rights being violated. A patient wanted to refuse all treatments, and the doctor declared him incompetent by employing the Baker Act The Baker Act states that the patient is mentally unstable and incapable of making rational decisions and, therefore, a danger to himself or herself. Under the Baker Act, the system can legally hold a patient for at least seventy-two hours, and only a psychiatrist can lift it. This patient was alert and cognitively aware of what he was doing at the time. He had not expressed any suicidal ideation. None of us could objectively discern why the physician made this decision. By taking this action, the physician stripped the patient of his legal rights, and he was therefore subjected to whatever decisions the doctor wanted to take on his behalf.

It seems at times that the Hippocratic Oath is merely reenacted for the sake of maintaining a tradition that goes back to the early 5th century B.C. In 1964, Louis Lasagna was said to have provided a modern version of the Hippocratic Oath. There are three statements in this oath that are worth mentioning (Lasagna 2016):

1. "I will apply, for the benefit of the sick, all measures which are required, avoiding…" the "traps of overtreatment…"

2. "I will remember that there is art to medicine as well as science, and that warmth, sympathy, and understanding may outweigh the surgeon's knife or the chemist's drug."

3. "I will not be ashamed to say 'I know not…'"

Let us analyze these statements:

"Applying all measures required for the benefit of the sick." Treatments and procedures are often implemented that do not benefit the patient. The trap of overtreatment frequently occurs, especially with the terminally ill, since they are often subjected to treatments that will not change the outcome of an illness. In fact, "…overtreatment and undertreatment occur, with adverse effects for patients" (Mamede and Schmidt 2014). My observations tell me that the error occurs more on the overtreatment side.

If "warmth, sympathy, and understanding" should prevail and, indeed, override a surgical procedure, or the use of another drug, then why are unnecessary surgeries performed or unnecessary drugs administered? It is your legal right to accept or deny all treatments, and it is your legal right to change your mind. I have taken care of patients on life support that were awake and fully aware of their condition, begging to be removed from life support. These patients had their wits about them to the extent that they would write out, *please let me go*.

Few physicians would be willing to say "'I know not…'" to their patients. Unfortunately, I have observed a highly honed art of dodging questions for which they have no answers. In most cases I believe that there is no any malintent. However, there are two things that will get patients and their family members angry: to be lied to, and to be misled. When this occurs the physician-patient trust is broken and the likelihood of litigation increases.

In most cases, however, these wishes were ignored by the family, the physicians, or both. Of course, the patients' clarity of mind and their understanding of their situation is usually brought into question; for example, "the patient is febrile or septic" or "the patient is in pain and simply stressed out." I have seen many patients fight for months until they came to terms with their condition. Once the inevitability of death was accepted, a mantle of peace seemed to have descended. They were finally at peace, and, in many cases, they started to enjoy life again with a heightened awareness of all things. My discussions with these patients were uplifting for I could see and feel that sense of inner peace and tranquility.

Due to the predicament in which many patients often find themselves, their mental and emotional states are often questioned. Questions are posed to patients that are either vague or ambiguous, and the same applies to some of the explanations provided. Individuals that are advanced in age may have some degree of dementia and forget certain things, such as who is the president of the United States or the month. The truth is, when you are that old, the president and the month often become irrelevant in one's life because that person has started to disengage from the mundane aspects of their existence. I have seen patients that did not know the current president, month, or the year but they knew their own name, place of birth, and their birthdate. Things that once mattered are no longer relevant. The focus is simply on living or letting go.

It is true, however, that the patient's cognitive abilities must be determined. Therefore, better questions should be created for those with advanced age, such as questions that are more relevant to the age group, in addition to the standard ones asked.

Another dilemma arises with the questioning process, and it has to do with the individual's cultural or ethnic background. In such cases, the questions should be posed by an individual from that culture or ethnic group or at least one that is familiar with the nuances of said culture. Using a wireless translation device on which a stranger asks questions is intimidating to some individuals, and they often fail to consider the nuances of the language. Their device translations are extremely concise, and that is not the way people normally communicate. I have served as a translator for many physicians, but I have always considered the distinctions of speech that allow for greater clarity during this process.

The examples of how a patient's wishes can be ignored are many, even when the patients have either clearly stated his or her wishes verbally, had DNR papers signed, or had an advance directive. Many times, it is the family members that demand that all things be done regardless of the patient's wishes. I have witnessed many physicians provide honest prognosis only to have the patient or family demand that everything be done. When that occurs, our hands are tied, and we perform our duties based on their wishes.

If you have a DNR, make sure that it is displayed in a prominent place at home such as on the refrigerator door (especially if you live alone) and make sure that you and your loved ones carry a legal copy. Unless you produce these documents, all medical personnel will be compelled, by law, to perform CPR, intubate you, and possibly place you on life support.

Patients often come to the emergency department and are placed on life support, including mechanical ventilation, for days or weeks, only to find out later that they had a DNR or advanced directive documents. The only alternatives at that point are to wait for possible improvement, the patient's demise, or the decision to remove mechanical ventilation.

When the decision must be made to remove life-support measures, the answers are wide-ranging. The advice will vary, but the following are quite common: *Let's wait a few days to see if the treatments are working*; *We just started the weaning process from the ventilator*; and, *Let's give it some time*. And, of course, *The patient's still alive, and the brain is still working*. These statements are fine if the possibility of a meaningful life exists. In such cases, it is a matter of waiting a long, agonizing period of time, filled with second-guesses and anguish.

These statements and other similar ones are often the sources of false hope. Being alive is a biological state of being that does not address the other dimensions of the individual. "The brain is still working" is a misleading statement for the same reasons because there is no reference to the mental, emotional, and spiritual capacities of the patient and their ability to lead a meaningful life. Sadly, the issues associated with the spiritual essence of the individual is never addressed or brought up in conversation.

One thing you must realize is that pain medications are often withheld for hours or days at a time, or not even given to the patient. You need to know that the patient can be sedated and still feel pain since it depends on the level of sedation being administered.

An intensive care nurse provided the following account regarding a patient that had advanced cancer, had surgery to remove a tumor, developed an infection, and was placed on life support. The patient's husband made it clear that they both knew the prognosis and that she did not want heroic measures. When asked about his wishes, he wanted his wife removed from the ventilator and all life support. However, the "…doctor said no. She said that the patient needed to complete the course of antibiotics to see if the infection could be cured, after which they could approach the question of whether to continue with intensive medical care. I imagine the doctor saw some distinction between letting the patient die of her primary, terminal diagnosis, and letting her die of a complication. So, the husband's efforts to stick up for his wife went unheard, and she stayed in the ICU, comatose, for about two more weeks—quite the opposite of her stated wish—before everyone agreed to let her go" (McConnell 2012).

❖

The following anecdote demonstrates the fact that many times, it is the family that prevents end-of-life wishes from being fulfilled:

> *Patient: Fictitious Name, Jane Suarez*
> *Age: 89*
>
> *Condition: End-stage COPD with other significant comorbidity factors such as cardiac arrhythmias and cancer.*

This patient was well known to the medical staff due to her many admissions throughout the years. Over the past few years, Mrs. Suarez's admissions became more frequent, and her breathing problems more pronounced and difficult to reverse. When I saw her during her last admission, I knew that she had embarked upon her final journey. Her daughter, unfortunately, could not come to terms with the reality of her situation, which was the fact that she was dying. She was a loving and caring daughter, but her denial of the facts prolonged her mother's death.

Mrs. Suarez ended up on life support and eventually underwent a tracheotomy. But even with a respirator, her breathing pattern remained the same. She exhibited a breathing pattern called *Cheyne Stokes* that usually precedes the end of life. It consists of periods of rapid to normal breathing, followed by periods of apnea or the cessation of respiration. This respiratory pattern is often referred to as the *death rattle* because secretions frequently accumulate in the back of the throat, thereby creating the congested or gurgling sound. This process is normal during the dying phase and does not indicate pain or suffering.

Regardless of all the signs of the approaching death, a few of us gently tried to get her daughter to think and acknowledge the reality of her mother's situation but to no avail. Eventually, her lifeforce failed, and we had to perform CPR on this frail eighty-nine-year-old woman! All because a family member refused to accept the uncontested truth that her mom was dying.

We all understand the anguish, the pain, and the doubts that often occur during such moments. We understand that it is difficult to let go of someone you love. But it was heart-wrenching to watch this frail woman who was actively dying, whose death was being prolonged through artificial means. In the end, no amount of heroic measures could remedy the outcome. The only solace would have been for her to die in peace instead of being thrust into the ambiguity of a technologically sustained life.

❖

In other cases, the dying process is prolonged even more because family members are not in agreement regarding the course of action on behalf of their loved one.

> *Patient: Fictitious name, Mrs. Smith*
> *Age: 75*
>
> *Condition: Respiratory Failure. Comorbidity factors included edema (excess fluid that accumulates in body cavities or tissues), ascites (the accumulation of fluids in the peritoneal cavity or abdomen), diffused bowel edema, sepsis, pneumonia, chronic diastolic heart failure (congestive heart failure), atrial fibrillation and atrial flutter, severe anemia, diabetes, COPD, hyperlipidemia (high cholesterol levels), hypertension, chronic liver disease, and an ex-smoker.*

The patient was placed on full life-support measures including feeding tubes, mechanical ventilation, antibiotics, blood pressure medications, arterial lines, central lines, Foley catheter, pain medications, insulin, sedatives, and more. We had tried to wean this patient off mechanical ventilation for close to two weeks, but she had failed every attempt. Her heart rate would go up, and respirations would also go up to unsustainable levels. Blood pressure would plummet as would her oxygen saturations, work of breathing would increase dramatically, and weaning parameters indicated an inability to wean. As a result, the patient needed to go to an LTAC (long-term acute care facility) for rehabilitation while on mechanical ventilation and possible weaning off vent. At this point, the patient needed a tracheotomy.

The insurance company wanted us to do a tracheotomy in the hospital and wait two more weeks to see if she could be weaned off the ventilator. If not, then they were considering paying for the LTAC facility. Other option: Perform a tracheotomy on the patient and send her to an SNF with minimal to nonexistent physical therapy or weaning off ventilator. (This second choice is what they were pushing for since it cost half of what the LTAC would cost.)

Question: Where in this scenario was the concern for this human being? This patient had entered her dying stage, however long it may have taken. The family had mixed feelings, and, from my interactions, they did not understand the reality of the situation.

Mrs. Smith failed multiple weaning attempts. After two weeks, the patient had to undergo a tracheotomy finally. Weaning attempts were continued post tracheotomy, since undergoing such a procedure often facilitates weaning. However, all attempts failed.

Finally, Mrs. Smith was transferred to an LTAC unit. She had been classified as ventilator-dependent, which refers to a patient that cannot be weaned off life support. One offspring was in favor of hospice and removing life support, but another offspring was adamant about continuing everything. The end result was that this patient was now confined to one of the many patient *warehouses* that, in some cases, serve to prolong the natural process of dying, such as the LTACs.

LTACs also provide the means for patients to recuperate from major catastrophic illnesses, but this is not always the case. I highly recommend that you visit such facilities and very carefully look around, ask questions, and look at the ratings. Do not allow yourself to be persuaded by the sales pitch and, instead, look at the facts. Physicians will often want the patient to go into a facility where they have privileges to practice. Continuity of care is usually advisable, but only if the facility the right one.

❖

Another source of anguish, for example, has to do with relationships between family members and the patient. These issues will extend beyond the family network and affect the nature and course of end-of-life decisions, as evidenced in the following anecdote:

I took care of an older woman (in her eighties) who ended up on mechanical ventilation and other life-support measures. This lady, whom we shall call Emily, had a DNR order which the offspring proceeded to cancel. Emily had clearly expressed that she did not want to continue living in her condition (she could not eat or drink due to poor swallowing function and the danger of aspiration), bedridden, and at the mercy of everyone else around her. She would beg for cold water, which we had to deny.

While she was on mechanical ventilation, she was fully alert and coherent. She would express to us her desire to be allowed to die. In the end, we managed to wean her off the mechanical ventilator, and she returned to her bedridden existence, one devoid of quality and meaningfulness. I took care of her after her sojourn in the intensive care unit. Her favorite term for me was "Honey."

There were times when I would hold her hand and try to comfort her while she begged me for a little "iced water." I would explain to her that the water could go into her lungs, making her very sick and that she could possibly die as a result. Her answer was always the same, *I don't care. I know what could happen. I just want a little bit of iced water.* It was heartbreaking to look into her eyes and hear her plea for peace.

Miss Emily was completely aware and could answer questions correctly. She was lucid but trapped in her own body. Every time I looked into her bright blue eyes, I could see the strength of character, her intelligence, and I would catch a glimpse of a very strong and independent woman. This particular case was medically successful in that we were able to extricate her from what could have turned out to be a prolonged stay on life support. This, however, has not deterred the march toward her departure from this earth.

I hope and pray that Miss Emily, that interesting lady with bright blue eyes, was able to finish her life in peace and tranquility. I hope that she does not find herself caught up in the net of our technological netherworld like so many others that die surrounded by cold machines and senseless procedures. I pray that Miss Emily will finally move on, peacefully, to a long-awaited spiritual reward!

Blurring the Line Between Life and Death

These occurrences are quite real, and they happen with greater frequency than you would imagine. At some point, the following question will come to mind, "What if the doctor is wrong about his or her prognostication?" *Any diagnosis or prognosis carries a margin of error, which is an occurrence that is not the physician's fault.* The variables are tremendous in terms of physical stamina, type of illness/es, the prior state of health, and the mental, emotional, and spiritual fortitude of the patient.

For example, I remember doing terminal extubation on a patient that had been on life support for quite a while. The family was fully prepared for the demise of their loved one once the ventilator was removed. Much to everyone's surprise, this patient did not die as quickly as expected. He was eventually transferred to the medical floor and subsequently to hospice care. The patient finally died about three months later.

Now, having kept this patient on life support would have only prolonged the inevitable outcome of his death. By removing life support and changing the status of this patient to comfort measures only (CMO), the patient's eventual passing was devoid of suffering, since the only medications that were given provided relief from pain and discomfort. These compassionate measures addressed the physical, mental, emotional, and spiritual concerns of the patient and family. To successfully address the end-of-life issues with the patient and family, they must have a clear understanding of the situation. This can be achieved regardless of cultural or ethnic background.

The following anecdote again reinforces the need for all of us to be well informed about our health or that of our loved ones. It also denotes the need for clear communication between patient, family, and the healthcare staff:

> Most of us rely on our personal beliefs, ethics, and morals when deciding what our loved ones would want. Trust your innate knowledge as well. At my urging, my mother had signed a living will and had advance directives stating that she did not want artificial hydration or nutrition. Due to the sudden onset of an illness, she was hospitalized for quite some time a few years ago. She was very confused, unable to coherently make her wishes known, and was refusing her liquid diet and medications. She had the ability to swallow but her medication-induced dementia prevented any oral intake. After over a week of IV hydration of saline (saltwater that provides no

caloric or nutrient intake), I insisted that a feeding tube be placed. Prior to hospitalization, she had been driving, doing her own cleaning and cooking, controlling her own bank account, shopping with friends, and otherwise enjoying a very active life for an octogenarian. I knew that she would continue to decline if nothing was done, and ultimately end up at "end of life" a lot sooner than she should have. The staff and physician argued that they must follow her advance directives even though I was her healthcare surrogate. After a few days of arguing, the tube was placed, and feeding was slowly begun. Ultimately, she went to rehab, began to eat again, had the feeding tube pulled then discharged to my sister's care for a few weeks. I am happy to report that as of this writing, she is nearly 87 and still living independently. If I had not persisted, I am quite sure she would have left us at the age of 82 (Duda 2017).

In this anecdote, the patient's condition had not turned irreversible, and life-support measures were properly applied.

This next anecdote illustrates how a properly applied life-support intervention can serve to bring peace and closure. The purpose was not to prolong the dying process of this patient but to give her the time she desired to be with her sisters one last time:

Another example of professional bias taught me a very valuable lesson. As a Nutrition Support professional, I was one who believed that heroic measures, including artificial nutrition and hydration, were not warranted with a terminal diagnosis. I received a call to evaluate a woman for the initiation of home parenteral nutrition.

She had terminal pancreatic cancer and was unable to tolerate the liquid food that was supposed to be infused through her feeding tube. She was extremely thin, with obvious signs of malnutrition. Her cancer treatments had been unsuccessful, all therapy (except the tube feeding) had been discontinued, and she was contemplating accepting hospice care. I asked her why she agreed to consider IV nutrition; what were her goals for the therapy? She said she just wanted to spend some quality time with her sisters. They had always made a week of shopping, talking, eating, and generally vacationing together, and she wanted to be with them again in a few weeks.

We continued talking while I completed my assessment. Internally I struggled with professional ethics versus personal morals. It slowly dawned on me that the only ethics that mattered were the ethics of the patient. We developed a plan, fed her through the medication port in her chest, and monitored her tolerance to the nutritional therapy. After about 2 weeks, she felt strong enough to enjoy the company of her sisters and told me that whatever I did, it was a miracle. I knew that after her family was gone and her last wish had been fulfilled, she would probably not last long. She was gone less than six weeks after our initial meeting. I think about her often and am proud that she changed me – my idea of what was moral and ethical. I believe that the soul knows the right thing to do, even though what we 'know' may be in opposition to what we have been taught (Duda 2017).

Modern technology has indeed blurred the line between life and death. The entire process is wrought with confusing and often opposing viewpoints, opinions, and information regarding death and dying. In the end, armed with the proper knowledge, you will be able to make the right decision either for yourself or someone you love. Without a clear understanding of the medical circumstances, you will be faced with a situation that could prolong the dying process of yourself or a loved one. When it comes to withholding artificial nutrition and hydration keep in mind that when:

> …artificial nutrition and hydration are withheld or withdrawn at the end of life; people do not die from starvation or thirst. Both families and medical personnel often find the withdrawal of treatment more emotionally difficult than the withholding of treatment, including artificial nutrition and hydration. But, legally and

ethically, there is no difference between the withholding or withdrawing of ANH at the request of a competent patient or authorized surrogate. Many studies have concluded that the underlying disease process is responsible for the person's death. Experts have shown that any discomfort experienced from thirst or hunger can be relieved with the provision of excellent mouth care, ice chips, and small bites of desired foods. After more than three decades providing nutritional therapies and observing countless individuals, I truly believe that when someone starts dying, they also stop eating. Don't be afraid to let your loved one progress to the other side. Remove your fears of letting go and trust our instinct. If you do, your decision will always be the right one (Duda 2017).

Definitions of Death

One of the issues that you will encounter that blurs the line between life and death, and is the direct result of modern technology is that there are various definitions of death (West's Encyclopedia of American Law 2016):

- *civil death* occurs when an individual is sentenced to life in prison thereby forfeiting his or her civil rights;

- *legal death* assumes that the individual has died (arises out of a prolonged absence);

- *natural death* refers to death by natural causes with no outside aid;

- *violent death* which is caused with the aid of an outside agency;

- *wrongful death* refers to a death which is willfully achieved or one that is caused by negligence

- *brain death* which refers to the cessation of all brain functions.

Science has advanced to such a degree that what was once a simple and natural process has now become a source of controversy and debate. We know by now that today's medicine can prolong life through artificial means such as mechanical ventilation, antibiotics, dialysis, and so much more. We also know that, in many cases, this has only served to prolong the process of dying rather than prolong the individual's life. The following excerpt will illustrate the point that I am trying to make (West's Encyclopedia of American Law 2016):

> Karen Ann Quinlan entered a comatose state, in 1975, and was put on life-support which included mechanical ventilation. Everything possible was done to no avail but the physicians refused to pronounce her case as 'hopeless.' Eventually, Karen's parents made the difficult decision of removing life-support while exempting the hospital and all staff from all responsibility. Nonetheless, the attending physician refused

their plea to end heroic measures. This forced Karen's parents to file a lawsuit to prevent the doctor from blocking the decisions taken on behalf of their daughter.

As a result of Karen Ann Quinlan's case, the court rulings changed the laws regarding a patient's rights to refuse heroic measures or for those legally recognized, such as next of kin:

> "In cases following Quinlan, courts have ruled that life-sustaining procedures such as artificial feeding and hydration are the legal equivalent of mechanical respirators and may be removed using the same standards" (Gray v. Romeo, 697 F. Supp. 580 [D.R.I. 1988]). Thankfully, the "...patient's legal right to refuse medical treatment has been grounded as well on the common-law right of bodily integrity, also called bodily self-determination, and on the liberty interest under the DUE PROCESS CLAUSE of the **Fourteenth Amendment**. These concepts are often collected under the term individual autonomy, or patient autonomy" (West's Encyclopedia of American Law 2016).

Modern scientific advances have succeeded in blurring the line between dying and living by thrusting an aspect of our humanity, our transiency, into the confusing world of semantics and legalese. In fact, we "...have opened a realm in which the distinction between life and death becomes blurred and contested—for clinical expertise, biomedical technologies, and hospital routines can sustain aspects of biological existence even when signs of a unique, valuable individual's life are absent or questionable" (S. R. Kaufman 2005).

We are bombarded through the media regarding all the wonderful and nearly miraculous medical tools and procedures. In the process, we are led to believe that medical science can see us through any critical illness. Thus, our expectations are extremely high (Bagshow, McDermid and Sean 2009). When discussing the issues of death and dying, it comes down to a matter of definition. The question then becomes: Which definition will you accept versus the definition favored by your physician?

Death is relatively simple to define since it is the cessation of all life-sustaining functions. It is a definition that creates an immense amount of sorrow and pain. Obviously, death itself will be delayed through the implementation of heroic measures. In the end, death will always claim its prize, but such delays are extremely costly on the physical, mental, emotional, spiritual, and financial levels. A great many people believe that "where there is life, there is hope." The question that begs to be asked is simple: What is the price paid for an extension of life?

Oftentimes, the heroic measures taken on behalf of a patient are futile, painful, costly, emotionally draining, and dehumanizing, regardless of what you may hear. The emotional part of ourselves will quite easily obscure our rational mind. When confronted with such situations, you may begin to hear and adhere to anything that represents the slightest fragment of hope, usually delivered by physicians and other healthcare workers.

A doctor will often deliver mixed messages that are devoid of any clarity regarding the real prognosis of the patient. What often occurs is that "…doctors err on the conservative side…" when making a diagnosis on the end of life (Fitzpatrick and Fitzpatrick 2010). What this means is that the physician will cautiously direct his or her dialogue toward a more positive outcome. Regardless of why a physician approaches end-of-life issues, the end result can adversely affect the decision-making process of the patient and his or her family.

Critically ill patients are usually under the care of several specialists. Among them are pulmonologists and intensivists, cardiologists, nephrologists, infectious disease specialists, oncologists, and an attending physician who can be the patient's family physician or one appointed by the hospital upon admission. What often occurs is that one or more physicians give a true prognosis, but another physician comes along and provides an opposing opinion or one that is, at best, vague.

The time of doctors coming together as a group to address the particular issues of a case is, for the most part, over. Discussions occur, but they are usually individual so that it is harder to reach a consensus. Doctors read physician notes, but these are condensed and limited to the immediate medical issues that are being addressed. Naturally, family members will hear and latch onto the statement that appears to be positive. However, "…the hope of a cure will always be shown to be ultimately false, and even the hope of relief too often turns to ashes" (Nuland 1995). It often happens that the physicians involved in a case are all in agreement regarding the patient's disease outcome, but the family insists on the continuation of life support.

What comes to mind is the story of the Greek Goddess of Dawn, Eos (also known as the Roman Goddess Aurora). Eos fell in love with a mortal man, the prince of Troy. The Goddess of Dawn went before Zeus and asked him to make her mortal lover immortal like her. Unfortunately, Eos forgot to ask Zeus to grant her lover eternal youth. Although her love for him never stopped, the prince of Troy continued to age and become extremely frail, endlessly suffering until he had lost his mind. Eos stayed away from him but continued to take care of him. In the end, the gods took pity on him and allowed him to finally die (GreekGods.Org - Mythology of Ancient Greece 2016).

The love that Eos felt was so great that, without realizing it, she had condemned the man that she loved, the prince of Troy, to a terrible fate of a prolonged death. Thus, decisions are often made with the best of intentions that turn out to be a nightmare, quickly turning into a scene from Dante's Inferno.

When patients and families insist on having everything done to prolong life (CPR, intubation, feeding tubes, medications, surgical procedures, tests, etc.), it becomes a waiting game to see if the family will finally accept the truth of the situation, or the patient mercifully dies sooner rather than later. When this occurs, the physicians have only two choices: remove themselves from the case or continue treating the patient per the family's request. The decision to initiate or continue life-support measures rests primarily in the hands of the patient, family, or both. Inform yourself and plan, and while doing so, consider the fact that you may be prolonging your suffering and death without any quality and meaningfulness or the prospect of having one.

As I have mentioned before, critical illnesses or conditions can occur at any time, regardless of age, economic status, area, religion, etc. We should all address these issues for ourselves and for our loved ones, including our children (as difficult as that may be).

I will never forget a patient that I took care of back in the mid-to-late 1970s. He was around thirty-four years of age and on life support, including a ventilator. This young man was contorted into a fetal position, trached (permanent tracheostomy tube), nothing but skin and bones, and in a persistent vegetative state. Seventeen years before, he had been in a terrible accident, and a medical error occurred that left him in this condition. His parents could not bear to remove him from life support.

This patient lived in the hospital because it was part of the legal settlement!

Accidents are not the only sources of such situations. Remember the cases of Terry Schiavo and Karen Ann Quinlan? These situations can come about unexpectedly.

In 2013, thirteen-year-old Jahi McMath underwent a tonsillectomy, a commonly performed surgical procedure to remove the patient's tonsils (two masses of tissue found on either side of the throat that are part of our immune system). The tonsils can get swollen and infected to a point in which they need to be removed, rarely leading to major complications. She was admitted to the intensive care unit, and eventually, Jahi went into cardiac arrest. Lack of oxygen to the brain left her braindead. Her mother felt that if her heart was beating that her child was still alive (Landau 2013).

We had a case in which a young man in his thirties had an anoxic event (lack of oxygen), which was long enough to cause irreversible brain damage. The lack of oxygen to the brain left him braindead. The patient's family member was reluctant to terminate life support, stating that, as long as his heart was beating, he was alive. Eventually, the family member agreed, and the patient died after being taken off life support.

I want you to know that a heart can be kept beating for a period of time outside of the body with the right fluids, chemicals, and oxygenation. I remember doing an experiment in high school biology that entailed keeping the heart of a frog beating for about thirty minutes outside the body. The experiment was successful, but was the frog alive?

Another incident occurred in 2016 involving a toddler, Israel Stinson. Israel was being treated for an asthma attack in early April when he suffered a cardiac arrest. More than likely, the cardiac arrest was secondary to an arrhythmia caused by a lack of oxygen. All of which resulted in brain death. Unfortunately, Israel is now confined to existence on life support. At best, this little boy will be in a persistent vegetative state (Sanchez 2016). This is an excellent example of the ambiguity caused by modern medical technology. Israel Stinson was kept alive through a life-support system, unable to live on his own. According to the reports, he was without oxygen for close to one hour (brain death begins after approximately six minutes without oxygen).

As you can see, the ages at which such tragedies occur are varied and unpredictable. As we get older, however, the likelihood of death overtaking us increases because of the wear and tear of the body, comorbidity factors, and the fact that the body is biologically hardwired to die. As we age, our bodies become less resilient, becoming harder and harder to recuperate from a devastating illness or accident.

Please understand that current medical science is truly wonderful, and it has gone a long way toward prolonging our lives. Today, intensive care units look like something out of a science fiction movie, due to the high-tech equipment and the chemical arsenal used to treat people. However, when all that technology is used to prolong the life of a patient that is dying, then this wonderful high-tech intensive care unit becomes "a high-tech torture chamber…" which provides a glimpse "…of hell during a person's last days on earth" (McConnell 2012).

A few years ago, I took care of a patient on mechanical ventilation who was in end-stage cirrhosis of the liver. The family was reluctant to terminate life-support measures, and the doctors had no choice but to comply with their wishes. Often, an individual with end-stage cirrhosis of the liver will die a very painful death which includes ascites (a large accumulation of fluid in the abdominal cavity), peritonitis (usually an inflammation caused by bacterial or viral infection in the abdominal cavity), encephalopathy (abnormal function of the brain), and generalized bleeding. This patient's abdomen was huge, and the skin was tight as a drum. Repeated attempts to drain the fluid were not successful since it would fill up again. Lungs were compromised, as was cardiac function, due to the complications of the disease. This went on for about three weeks until the patient finally died by bleeding out through every orifice in the body.

What kept this patient alive for so long was the life support prolonging his death. This was a horrible image to have of a loved one at the end of their life!

Those patients that survive long enough will generally be transported to an LTAC. Usually, the reasoning behind this is that the patient will need more time on mechanical ventilation and intensive rehabilitation. Often, this occurs because the insurance company's allotted coverage for an acute care facility is about to run out, or it has already run out. Other provisions in the insurance coverage will take over once the patient has been transferred so that their stay at the LTAC will be covered. Eventually, regular hospital funding starts again, and a revolving-door process starts.

If you do not have insurance, then you will be stuck in limbo or placed in a nursing home, since most places will not take you unless you have coverage.

We currently have two cases in which placement has been a nightmare. Both patients are on life support, and both underwent tracheotomies. They are both neurologically compromised. One patient does not have insurance, and the other patient's insurance does not cover long-term care. In any event, upwards of ninety facilities within a one-hundred-mile radius have been contacted. All refused to take the patients for various reasons, including "not enough personnel" to handle the care of the patient. This often occurs regardless of health insurance coverage.

In the meantime, both patients are awaiting placement if they can find some government coverage. I see many case managers scrambling to find placement for an uninsured patient, for they are under tremendous pressure from the administration. Some type of minimal government funding is usually allocated with limited coverage. As a result, many patients will end up in facilities that are less than desirable.

The facilities that eventually take such patients are often depressing and frequently in a deplorable state. To make matters worse, most of these facilities are seriously understaffed. Many are riddled with various drug-resistant organisms, and the staff is seriously overworked because of poor patient-to-healthcare-worker ratios.

To illustrate, one respiratory therapist may be responsible for six or more seriously ill patients on mechanical ventilation with multiple medical conditions. You must wonder how they can get away with such things! Is regulatory enforcement so poor, or do they simply turn a blind eye? But there are enormous financial incentives "'…built into the programs that most often serve people with advanced serious illnesses—Medicare and Medicaid—encourage providers to render more services and more intensive services that are necessary or beneficial,' …according to Dying in America, a massive report issued in September by the Institute of Medicine" (Whoriskey 2014). Rest assured that there is a definite interest in money, and, the greater the acuity (refers to the severity of an illness), the greater the charge.

Many physicians are against using our technology to prolong the dying process, thereby prolonging the suffering that the patient and family experience. One critical care physician made the following statement: "'I'm running a warehouse for the dying...'" and of the "ten patients in her unit, she said, only two were likely to leave the hospital for any length of time" (A. Gawande 2014).

The conditions in which these patients find themselves are referred to as the "'greenhouse effect,' since, like plants in the winter, they cannot survive outside of the life-sustaining greenhouse of the ICU. They are often consigned for weeks or even months to a sort of medical purgatory, attached by tubes in their tracheas to ventilators, with catheters protruding from their necks, chests, abdomens or bladders. When awake, they are in constant discomfort, chronically deprived of sleep, and stripped of any dignity..." (Breslow 2015).

Numerous conditions lead to the process of dying. But, as I have said before, modern medical technology often prolongs the process of dying rather than the process of living. The issue is controversial from a medical and legal perspective, as well as from that of the patient and family.

For instance, "The Society of Critical Care Medicine defines therapeutic futility as treatment that 'does not accomplish its intended goal, that is, beneficial physiologic effect'" (Bagshow, McDermid and Sean 2009). Then why are patients subjected to countless treatments that do not accomplish anything other than prolonging the process of dying? In addition, "The

American Thoracic Society statement on Withdrawing and Withholding Life Sustaining Therapy defines futility as the combination of two criteria, 1) lack of medical efficacy, as judged by the patient's physician, and 2) lack of a meaningful survival, as judged by the personal values of the patient" (Bagshow, McDermid and Sean 2009).

Please note that the physician is at liberty to order any treatment if he or she thinks that it will be beneficial to the patient, and that is to be expected. It is also very easy for the physician to persuade a patient and family members to accept the treatments proposed since they are in control of the situation and because they are seen as figures of authority. It is very easy for a physician, or other medical personnel, to befuddle your mind with the medical and technical jargon, and not everyone is adept at translating that technical terminology. It is up to the patient and/or the family to make sure that they have a clear understanding of the facts. It may be helpful to focus your attention on the following issues: possible treatments (including their aim, potential adverse reactions or complications, short and long-term side effects, and actual impact on the underlying issues), prognosis, and, most importantly, the effects on your life that can be expected should a certain course of action be accepted.

Dr. Jeff Gordon wrote that today's "high-tech medical care can sustain technical life—the beating heart—but utterly fails to restore real quality of life for many. There comes a point when physicians can prolong dying, but not provide quality living" (Brody 2009). Our life-extending procedures often end up putting the patient and family through the horror of watching a loved one die a very slow and often agonizing death. You could argue that the patient is provided with pain medication and sedation, but that is not always the case since patients are given sedation vacations to allow them to wake up, and pain medications are often withheld for weaning purposes.

Recently, I took care of a woman on life support. She was on mechanical ventilation, had chest tubes on either side of her chest, urine catheter, intravenous catheters, tracheostomy tube, developed subcutaneous emphysema (trapped air underneath the skin) around her upper chest, and was on a multitude of drugs. She also had multiple procedures involving radiology and a few surgical procedures.

We tried to wean her off mechanical ventilation utilizing different approaches. She would tolerate the weaning procedures for a while, but in the end, she failed the trials. This woman was off sedation almost the entire time and sporadically received pain medication. She was awake, and we could see her expressions of anguish and extreme discomfort. Sometimes she would look at us with a heartbreaking expression. After several weeks of this technological limbo, her daughter came in and had her extubated. Finally, hospice was called; she survived until the following day.

If the patient is comatose, we are taught that they are unlikely to feel pain, but they also teach us that the ability to hear is the last thing to go! And let us not forget the spiritual aspects of this situation.

To those of you contemplating doing everything that can be done, whether out of love, remorse, or a lack of understanding, or both, I would like you to remember the mythological story of the Greek Goddess Eos and what became of the man she so dearly loved. One crucial element in your decisions is that of demanding the unadulterated truth, especially the truth concerning the eventual course of the illness. Do not be fooled by unrealistic expectations. Please open your mind, your heart, and your eyes, and truly see what is before you. Become *aware*. Remember that the truth, however painful, is better than the dangling carrot of false hopes, which will, inevitably, be snatched away.

ೞ ೲ

God offers to every mind its choice
between truth and repose.
Take which you please,
you can never have both.

Ralph Waldo Emerson (1803-1882)
U.S. poet, essayist, and lecturer

CHAPTER FOUR

Telling the Truth

Tell the truth to a dying patient and his or her family, is a huge and complex topic of controversy. You might think that communication with patients and family members would be easy when compared to the complexities of medical treatments. But I have witnessed, time and time again, the inadequacies in the interaction between medical professionals, patients, and family.

We are born, we live our lives, and then we die. *Dying is not an illness that can be cured or a malfunction that can be repaired.* However, we tend to complicate everything by thinking and rethinking, and then we put it into the framework of science in such a way that it will provide us with the sense of being in control, however fleeting that may be. We try to rationalize everything into nice little packages designed to be more acceptable to our sensibilities. It is a way of coping with our mortality.

Regardless of the reasons, most people will instinctively shy away from the topic of death and make it taboo (a subject that is forbidden). As natural as death and dying are, they remain sensitive subjects, since they have a definite impact on the patient, family, and significant other. It is further complicated because of our modern technology, which has blurred the definition of *terminal illness* and the patient's *prognosis*.

Terminal—A Confusing Term

Terminally ill refers to any disease or condition that is progressive, irreversible, and that will ultimately end with death. Terminal illnesses and conditions are prolonged because of our medical interventions. The term *terminal* is no longer clearly defined. At what point in time does a patient become terminally ill? It is inconceivable to many individuals that a person in their eighties, nineties, or beyond should be considered as being *terminal* due to their apparent health. However, the body has continued to deteriorate; its ability to repair itself is no longer what it used to be, and, eventually, one or more of the body's systems will fail.

Regardless of this knowledge, it seems that medical science insists on prolonging life at the expense of dignity and quality. In my experience, a patient's terminal stage can be prolonged for weeks, months, and even years, depending on the individual case and circumstances. I am not opposed to prolonging life provided that we are not prolonging the process of dying.

To prolong the dying process is cruel and inhumane. *Let there be no misunderstanding. I do not support euthanasia (assisted death) or any other form of suicide. I do support, however, allowing one to die with dignity and respect when their time comes, and according to their wishes.*

Prolonging Life vs. Quality of Life

It is indeed cruel to dangle the carrot of hope in front of those that are dying. The ambiguities that surround the term *terminal* complicate the decision-making process of patients and families, as well as the administration of health-related care. These issues also impact the actual projection or natural progression of a disease or illness, since it will be altered by employing life-support measures. The truth of the matter is that medical science is not an exact science, as the medical profession would often have us believe. The reason why I make this statement is simple. Each patient is different, and this impacts the way the body responds to disease processes.

Patients with the same disease react differently and have different capabilities in terms of their physical, mental, emotional, and spiritual stamina. When a person enters the dying phase, it will take its natural course unless we interfere with it. What remains unchanged, however, is that the person is dying. The pace of death is the only thing that's changed.

By keeping the patient and family uninformed as to the reality of the expected outcome, the physician and the rest of the medical establishment have, unintentionally, robbed them of valuable information that could empower them to "…put their affairs in order…" including "…making decisions about end-of-life care, finances, guardianship, power of attorney, and where to die" (Lowry 2013). It also could provide the patient and family time to adjust to the reality of the prognosis, rather than to embrace false hopes only to have them dashed to pieces when reality dawns.

We need to accept our fleeting nature and forgo ego and pride. We are not all-powerful, and death will be our unerring companion. Learning the truth, however difficult, preserves your autonomy, or your ability to govern yourself, and preserves your freedom and right of self-determination.

Unfortunately, many terminally ill patients are not fully informed. "A recent American study showed that 69% of 710 patients with incurable lung cancer and 81% of 483 patients with colorectal cancer who received palliative chemotherapy were unaware that the treatment was not curative (N Engl J Med. 2012; 367:1616-1625)" (Lowry 2013).

In simpler terms, 490 patients with incurable lung cancer and 391 patients with colorectal cancer had no idea that the treatments being given to them would not cure them! Besides, most chemotherapy treatments make the patients feel miserable. The side effects of chemotherapy can include any of the following: fatigue, pain (headaches, muscle pains, nerve pains, stomach pains), mouth and throat sores, diarrhea, nausea and vomiting, constipation, blood disorders (low white blood cell count, leaving you vulnerable to infections; low red blood cell count, anemia; low platelets, leaving you prone to bleeding), nervous system effects, changes in thinking and memory, sexual and reproductive problems, loss of appetite, hair loss, and, finally, permanent damage to different organs (American Society of Clinical Oncology (ASCO) 2005-2016).

Prior to my mother's death, she had developed mediastinal cancer. "The mediastinum is the part of the chest that lies between the sternum and the spinal column, and between the lungs. This area contains the heart, large blood vessels, windpipe (trachea), thymus gland, esophagus, and connective tissues" (Yi-Bin 2014). The usual treatment would have been chemotherapy since the tumor was inoperable. An oncologist was called in, and of course, he offered *palliative treatments for the cancer.*

Successful treatment rates drastically decrease for "…most cancers that have metastasized (spread beyond the original cancer site), chemotherapy cannot cure the cancer. However, chemotherapy may be helpful in shrinking the cancer, improving or completely eliminating distressing symptoms caused by the cancer for a period of time and helping you live longer. The use of chemotherapy in these situations is called *palliative chemotherapy*" (Center to Advance Palliative Care 2014).

Unfortunately, the oncologist had given my sister a fragile thread of hope and a sense of false optimism that the chemotherapy would change the outcome. This was not done out of malice. It is simply the way that he was trained and an example of the current approach to dealing with terminally ill patients. Such statements, unfortunately, are given without consideration of the mental and emotional impact it may have on the patient and family.

As a result, this issue caused my sister quite a bit of distress. Not fully understanding the implications of this "palliative chemotherapy," she thought that our mother's condition would improve. It took me quite a while to convince her that chemotherapy would have only made our mother's last days incredibly miserable. That change in outcome would have been a few extra weeks of life (at best) while suffering from the side effects of the chemotherapy! The doctor meant well but remember that the "road to hell is paved with good intentions." My mother did not want to go through such extremes and, besides, she was ready to go on to the next life where she knew that my dad and other members of the family were waiting for her.

Eventually, we took our mother home with hospice services, and a few weeks later she passed away very peacefully, surrounded by her children, grandchildren, and great-grandchildren.

Telling the Truth in a Multicultural Environment

Telling the truth to a terminally ill patient is complicated by cultural and ethnic backgrounds. To illustrate, Japanese patients, Ethiopian patients, and patients from Saudi Arabia feel that the information "…belongs to the family, who then use the information in the best interests of the patient" (O'Kelly, et al. 2011). In some cases, such as in the Muslim culture, "…it is God who permits death, hence giving up hope is against religious teaching, amounting to a loss of faith in God" (H. F. Wolcott 1991). Also, many Spanish families feel that it is their duty, not the doctor's, to inform the patient.

Family members will often withhold disclosing the true essence of the condition because they fear that revealing the information will be detrimental to their loved one. There is a degree of wisdom associated with this perspective since a state of depression and anxiety can lower the person's immune system that could then cause a much more rapid progression of the disease. But assuming that telling the truth will be detrimental is depriving the patient of his or her autonomy in deciding how to manage the end of life.

I remember many years ago, being present in a hospital room when a doctor came in to deliver a diagnosis of terminal cancer. This patient, in her mid-forties, was silent and calm as she listened to the physician's prognosis. Naturally, he recommended chemotherapy and radiation therapy, but she refused. He then asked her why? And her response was that she knew that she would not die from this illness (this patient had undergone exploratory surgery, and they closed her up because her cancer was so widespread that they could not do anything for her). I had the pleasure of watching this patient walk out of the hospital free of cancer after having been thoroughly re-examined!

When we questioned the doctor, he was upset and said that it was just a matter of spontaneous remission or a miracle. I firmly believe that being aware of her prognostication led this patient to heal. Whether it was spontaneous remission, a miracle, mind over matter, or a combination of these, we will never know. Just because the overall tendency of a culture is to withhold information from the dying does not mean that every individual in that culture feels or thinks the same way. What we should keep in mind is that many individuals come to terms with death and dying and actually improve their quality of life at the end.

As healthcare workers, we must all respect cultural variations regarding truth-telling to the terminally ill. Violating this will increase the emotional distress felt by the patient and the family. Culture is, fundamentally, the driving force that shapes an individual's propriospect.

Anthropologist Ward H. Goodenough coined the term propriospect. Goodenough proposed, "…that each of us develops a unique way of thinking, a personal culture, that he labeled a 'propriospect.' The term refers to each individual's highly subjective and personal view of the world" (H. Wolcott 2008). You must keep in mind that the physicians will have their unique way of viewing the world, which, in the end, will influence their decisions even while trying to maintain scientific impartiality. Even while observing and respecting cultural preferences regarding truth-telling, the physician should tell the truth to the patient's family and significant other. What family members and patients do with that truth is up to them, but at least the medical establishment complied with what can only be called a moral imperative.

It is interesting to note that, in most cases, the terminally ill patient is aware that they are nearing the end of life. And yet, everyone concerned will enact this play during which the main issue is *known* to everyone, but it is never mentioned. I have experienced this *cultural dance* with my own family.

When my father entered the phase of actively dying, he, unfortunately, ended up being intubated and put on mechanical ventilation for a couple of days. We all knew the reality of the situation, but it was never spoken out loud. As a respiratory therapist, I knew what was going on, but I never said a word until the very end. I chose to give the rest of the family time to come to terms. I limited myself to relaying the information given to me by the physician because I was the spokesperson for the family. My father was aware of his dying, even though he had advanced Alzheimer's. There were times when he was quite lucid, and he would ask me to make sure to take care of my mother.

My mother also knew that she was dying, but she never said it out loud. We all knew that her end was approaching, but it was never verbalized. Discussions regarding the reality of her medical state were kept among the family members. I share with you a few of her final words that expressed her free spirit and yearning to exit her frail, immobile body in which she felt trapped. She looked at me and said, *I want to dance and fly!*

Withholding the Truth

Regardless of how the truth is or is not presented, the person that is terminally ill will usually know that they are dying. It could be due "…to popular belief, or perhaps from wishful thinking—because of our own discomfort with death—dying people know they are dying" (Kelley 1992). We all have an ability that allows us to *know* something. It is experienced spontaneously and in different settings. It is a knowledge that is derived from the person's *inner* or spiritual self, as well as from experience. When this occurs, one "…knows something directly that could not possibly be known in any other way…" and this *knowing* "…is subjective and private, and it is tremendously significant" (W. C. Tremmel 1976). When this *knowing* occurs it is not generally perceived by everyone, not "…because one person's faculty of knowing extends wider than that of another but because those common notions are opposed to the prejudiced opinions of some people who, consequently, cannot easily grasp them, even though other people who have been liberated from those prejudices perceive them very clearly" (Descartes 2003).

This *knowing*, when it occurs, is either shared with other family members or not. When the patient opts to keep quiet about their *knowing*, it is usually to protect those that they love. However, withholding the truth from a dying patient is oftentimes a game of self-deception, since the individuals concealing the information assume that the patient does not have a clue as to what is going on! Remember the lie detector.

To those in the field of medicine, allow me to remind you that most of the world has become multicultural because of modern technology and rapid means of transportation. Therefore, most cultures throughout the world will encounter other cultures and their perspectives regarding health, healing, religion and other belief systems. Religious beliefs will have a definite impact on how individuals perceive their end of life.

For example, "...the patients' and their families' trust in God may deter them from making decisions about life and death. Their reluctance to talk and accept a fatal diagnosis means they are often unwilling to consider forgoing life-prolonging/sustaining futile treatment" (O'Kelly, et al. 2011). These failures to discuss such critical issues could very well lead to a prolonged death within the confines of a technological nightmare.

Withholding the truth for whatever reason will, in most cases, prompt the patient or family to opt for heroic measures under the misguided belief that recovery and return to the previous level of quality is possible. Sadly, the dying patient's quality of life will significantly deteriorate. Research has shown that end-of-life "…discussions are associated with less aggressive medical care near death and earlier hospice referrals. Aggressive care is associated with worse patient quality of life and worse bereavement adjustment" (Wright, Zhang and Ray 2008).

Consequences of Withholding the Truth

Perhaps it is time to ask ourselves the following question: *What is the definition of bad news?* We all know unwelcome news refers to something unpleasant and, therefore, undesirable. Thus, the delivery of shocking news can be awkward and difficult. Physicians, being human, often find it difficult to deliver unwelcome news, and this can often result in subjecting patients "…to harsh treatments beyond the point where treatment may be expected to be helpful" (Baile 2000). When facing the undeniable reality that a patient is dying, doctors are often advised to avoid statements such as: there "…is nothing more we can do for you" (Baile 2000). Avoiding such statements leaves the door wide open to interpretation.

The following anecdote, provided by an excellent and compassionate nurse, illustrates what could easily occur when we withhold the truth from a patient:

> I took care of this young man who was extremely septic. The surgeons kept cutting or amputating parts of his legs-knowing that he was not going to recover. One surgeon finally said, *you know you are going to die*. After the surgeon left, the patient said to me, *why didn't you tell me that I was going to die?* It was one of the worst feelings because I felt like I had withheld information that would have helped him make decisions about what to do for the remaining days of his life.

By sidestepping such assertions, the patient and family may easily conclude that there *is* something more that can be done. What matters most is how the information is delivered. Is it cold and detached, or is there some degree of genuine compassion?

You can provide such a proclamation while at the same time letting the patient know that there are comfort measures that can be implemented. Not telling the truth will also undermine any trust established between the patient and the doctor. Honesty on the part of the physician is essential regardless of how difficult the subject! As healthcare workers, we require the truth from our patients for us to improve the treatment process. Patients and family members are interrogated regarding their personal lives. This is necessary if we are to obtain a clear and accurate picture of the patient's state of health, both past and present. The least that the medical establishment can do is honor the patient and family members with the truth. Withholding the truth from patients and family members is detrimental. Regardless of cultural and ethnic differences, truth-telling to the patient and family is an act of respect.

"Without the disclosure of truth to the dying patient, individuals are likely to be subjected to aggressive treatments which will turn their dying into a painful, expensive and dehumanizing process" (Drane 2002). As human beings, we relate to each other in some way, shape, or form. One of the aspects of human relationships that allows for prolonged interpersonal relationships is that of honesty. When honesty is lacking or missing, the relationship begins to fall apart.

Also, lying is reprehensible, amoral, and considered a sin in many religions. Lying to patients and family members is viewed as an act of betrayal from the medical establishment, which elicits feelings of distrust and anger. Such emotional states are not conducive to harmony or acceptance and are harmful to the patient.

Professional medical associations have addressed the ethical aspects of truth-telling: "The Code of the American Nurses Association states: 'Clients have a moral right…to be given accurate information.' It urges nurses to avoid false claims and deception. Even the 'Principles of Medical Ethics' of the American Medical Association, in 1980, included a reference to honesty. 'A physician shall deal honestly with patients and colleagues and strive to expose those physicians deficient in character or competence, or who engage in fraud or deception'" (Drane 2002). However, *accurate* information and *honesty* are terms that are stretched and skewed on a day-to-day basis.

Unfortunately, a very large number of physicians are reluctant to expose those colleagues with questionable competence. I know this to be true, for I have seen it throughout my career. In any event, the medical staff, including the physicians, can be quite selective when it comes to telling the truth, especially in cases where the prognosis is not favorable. What often occurs is a mental dance between the hospital personnel, the patient, and the family. The issues are artfully circumvented without outright lying, although the omission of the truth is a lie!

Patients and family members will often question healthcare workers regarding their condition. What often happens, however, is that they are told to talk to the doctor. In these situations, a family liaison is usually appointed and is responsible for conveying the truth, in some fashion, to the patient, family, and friends. Keep in mind that, without malice, the contact person may *selectively* provide unpleasant information in a positive way, thereby misleading both the patient and family. The results can be devastating.

I have also witnessed selective truth-telling on numerous occasions by various members of the healthcare team. The medical issues with a critically ill and dying patient are complex since they usually involve several organ systems and infectious processes. During the time that the patient is in the intensive care unit, you will observe a roller coaster effect associated with systems; such as the heart and circulation, kidneys, skin, intestines, liver, etc.

For instance, most infections can be treated, blood pressure can be stabilized, fluid retention can often be controlled through drugs, and cardiac arrhythmias can often be managed with medications. So, the infectious disease specialist will report that the infection is gone, and lab tests are back to normal or improving. The cardiologist can report that the arrhythmias and blood pressure are now under control, and the nephrologist (kidney specialist) can report that fluid retention is going down, the kidneys are now working again, or that the problem can be corrected through dialysis. Once again, what the patient or family may hear is that an improvement has occurred.

In the meantime, the family will be grasping for those elusive rays of hope, such as that new drug, procedure, or miracle that will restore their loved one to health. Yet, the patient is still dying or suffering a worse fate, whether it is from cancer, chronic congestive heart failure, brain damage that leads to a persistent vegetative state, end-stage COPD or any number of conditions that are progressive, irreversible, and ultimately terminal.

These therapies and interventions prolong the process of dying or provide short-lived advances that loved ones perceive as *real* improvements. In the end, a panoply of drugs is used, since more medications are prescribed to counteract the adverse effects of the other medicines, and the cycle continues. The medical staff should not assume that the patient or family will have a clear grasp of the gravity of the situation; otherwise, this will lead to a communication failure.

Communication Failure

There are several factors associated with communication failure (Meier 2006):

"Knowledge gap"

The prognosis of terminal illness may be obvious to the medical professionals but not to the family. Selectively providing truthful information without addressing the overall negative prognosis of the patient is "…a major source of misunderstanding, mistrust and compounded suffering for all concerned."

"Transference and countertransference"

When confronting the nonmanipulable reality of our mortality, individuals, regardless of educational background or socioeconomic status, will see the physician as someone with almost god-like powers and abilities to heal. This is called transference (the individuals transfer their own perceptions to another person; in this case, the physician). In turn, the physician

---

will experience countertransference. When this occurs, the doctors will "…unconsciously want to be forgiven for the patient's bad outcome; they personalize and cannot bear the…" family's "…disappointment and rage, normal and understandable as those actions are."

"Physician discomfort with bad outcomes"

Our society has been imbued with the idea that through our technology, illnesses and even death can be conquered. This mindset not only permeates healthcare education, but is found any place where health care is practiced. However, the "…inconvenient truth is that every patient will sicken and die, and it is beyond our power…to prevent it."

"Lack of education in how to approach the care of the seriously ill and their families"

These skills exist and can be easily taught to all healthcare personnel.

❖

I truly believe that most medical workers care for the wellbeing of the patient and their family or significant other. Yet, we are all restrained because of our current healthcare mentality in which the patient is no longer a patient but a client.

Catering to patients as if they were clients in a hotel often results in increased tension and decreases the interactions between patients and staff. Many patients take advantage of this mindset and become very demanding, often refusing to do things for themselves that they could otherwise do. As a result, the exchange of information often decreases for fear of upsetting the patient.

Thus, all healthcare professionals must exercise caution, not for the sake of avoiding unnecessary hurt but to appease the patient or family. Since telling the truth could cause distress (even though that truth will, in the end, help you to make the right decisions), you will be less likely to receive the whole truth! There is no secret formula to decrease the level of distress caused by being told the truth. It depends on each individual's propriospect, level of education, belief system, and mental and emotional balance. All of these aspects, combined, form the person's ability to cope with various situations.

Patient Satisfaction and How It Impacts Insurance Reimbursement

Like any other business, patient satisfaction is of utmost importance, since it directly impacts reimbursement from insurance companies. As of October 1, 2012, a portion of the hospital's reimbursement became dependent on patient satisfaction (not necessarily associated with positive medical outcomes). As a matter of fact, thirty "percent of the program's financial incentive is based on how well hospitals score on patient satisfaction, as measured by the Hospital Consumer Assessment of Healthcare Providers and Systems (HCAHPS) survey" (Guadagnino 2012). Unfortunately, this creates an unhealthy atmosphere in which highly skilled professionals are perceived as nothing more than highly paid servants by some patients. An enormous amount of time is spent on averting unfavorable reports from the patient and family, a lot of which has nothing to do with the medical care involved.

To make matters worse, hospitals, regardless of what they may say or advertise, often run their shifts without the appropriate patient-to-healthcare-worker ratios. So, instead of utilizing the amazing talent and dedication found within a hospital for the sole purpose of taking care of the sick, much of that talent is misused for the sake of a satisfaction survey or the bottom line!

True healers, whether they be doctors, nurses, or therapists, provide much more than their expertise in the various fields of medicine. A true *healer* is one that addresses not just the needs of the physical body but the mental, emotional, and spiritual dimensions.

Unfortunately, "…measuring and rewarding 'patient satisfaction' isn't translating into good medical care. A patient who is highly satisfied with, say, the amount of pastrami on his lunchtime sandwich may still be dead in an hour" (Kenen 2015). Joanne Kenen (Kenen 2015) states that out of thousands of hospitals surveyed, two-thirds of hospitals with the lowest outcome scores on the highest number of deaths, readmissions, and serious complications scored higher because of their patient satisfaction score! These surveys were created for the industry and consumerism, and, as a result, they lack humanism.

Actual Outcome Scores: The Things That Matter the Most

Allow me to borrow an old saying, *Caveat Emptor*, buyer beware! If you are looking for a hospital, then investigate actual outcome scores—the things that matter the most: number of nosocomial infections (hospital-acquired infections), surgical outcomes, mortality rates for various diseases, etc. Regardless of where you decide to go, it is ultimately up to you to make sure that you are being presented with the truth. You have the legal right to know the truth, to refuse or accept treatment, and to change your mind at any time.

Trust the medical team, but do not imbue them with idealistic powers and abilities. They are human. Make sure that your anticipations are realistic and not based on fantasy. Remember, it is up to the patient and family to maintain all communication channels open with the healthcare staff. Please avoid taking your frustrations and anger out on them. They are not your maids and butlers, so do not treat them as servants. The hospital staff members are highly trained and dedicated individuals diligently working on your behalf. Please do not touch any of the equipment and do not get in the way while they are taking care of your loved one. Ask only important questions, and do not question them incessantly. Of utmost importance, be grateful to all of them and let them know.

Progress is constantly being made through scientific research, and, yes, unexplained recoveries have occurred. But, how long will you wait while your loved one is dying a piece at a time, and how long will you wait while your family member suffers a long and prolonged death?

I encourage you to read and re-read this book and arm yourself with this information. I implore you to think. How would you feel if you or a loved one were consigned to seemingly unending suffering in this techno-hell? Remember that, aside from the physical suffering, the spirit is also caught in what could be called a state of Medical Limbo, described as a stagnant, nonmanipulable existence filled with uncertainty. That spirit is caught between this world and the next. Thus, the next question to ponder should be, *Do I hold on, or do I let go?*

ೞ ೱ

*There is no worse lie than a truth misunderstood
by those who hear it.*

William James, Lectures XIV and XV, "The Value of
Saintliness," The Varieties of Religious Experience

CЗ Юつ

True love doesn't have a happy ending,
because true love never ends.
Letting go is one way of saying I love you.

Unknown

CHAPTER FIVE

Holding On or Letting Go

Two universal truths are the source of so much suffering: *attachments* (think of it as a bond, connection, link, or tie that is created) and *unrealistic expectations*. We form bonds to ideas, ideologies, sex, money, jobs, or professions, a particular philosophy, life, people, and just about everything you can think of in this world. These connections are a great source of sorrow since they are all ephemeral. Impractical hopes will greatly increase the degree of misery, for they are not based on reality. Common sources of suffering are the associations that we form with other individuals in our life and the unrealistic expectation that they will be around forever.

Nineska M. del Rosario, M.A., C.R.S, while discussing the contents of this book, mentioned to me that she "…had seen people in counseling that were having difficulties with family members not trying to solve their differences on the idea that they would be around forever." We abhor the notion that someone that we love may die. I believe that we are all subconsciously aware of our own mortality. Nevertheless, due to the transient nature of our existence, we try to anchor ourselves to this world and this reality by forming connections to numerous things.

These attachments occur in many ways and to various degrees. Powerful ties are created regarding life and its physical pleasures. Emotions, such as those associated with love, anger, greed, hatred, resentments, concerns, etc., are also quite common. You can also form strong links to success, power, and life, as well as a philosophy or religion.

Many attachments are combined, and these can become very powerful. For instance, you can become attached to your childhood home and the memories associated with that period. You can also form associations to simple objects associated with the memories of past or present family members. These ties may involve anything such as clothing, jewelry, pictures, decorations, kitchen implements, and tools, to name a few. You may also be attached to the emotions elicited from such objects since they serve to bring up pleasant (or unpleasant) memories. Such steadfast ties can also keep you living in the past, while expectations can keep you focused on the future. The result is that you stop living, for living occurs in the present, in the here-and-now!

Many attachments are minor ones, and others are transient. Some, however, are so deeply rooted within us that we find it difficult to let go even when facing the end of life. Now, the overall effects of some powerful bonds are often exponentially increased, depending on the set of anticipations that are associated with a particular attachment. The more unlikely the expectation, the harder it will be to let go of an attachment. These bindings that we create, and their accompanying expectations, vary depending on the individuals' view of the world.

To further complicate matters, these attachments and ephemeral anticipations are often created and fueled by the cultural environment in which we live. And, most importantly, we form strong, deep-rooted bonds to our relationships and the individuals involved. These individuals could be family members, boyfriends, girlfriends, lovers, husbands, wives, children, friends, and even pets. Normally, we form extremely powerful bonds within our nuclear and extended family members, friends, and lovers.

These attachments and expectations create an enormous amount of suffering for all of us! You may ask, Why? The answer is rather simple (or so it seems). The one constant in this universe is that everything changes: our bodies, cellular structure, our health, our way of thinking, our feelings, our ideas, philosophies, beliefs, and on, and on! The best that we can hope for is that the changes that do occur are on a parallel course or are improvements.

However, this is not what we are led to believe because our society is quite adept at creating illusions. Thus, our culture creates the illusion that we can become ageless, and that all illnesses can be conquered, as well as our mortality. The truth is, "…that, despite the promises of technology, human frailty in the presence of death has ultimately changed very little. The faith that Americans place in science and technology, however, has instilled unworkable anticipations of control within the American frame of mind. The result of these expectations is that feelings of powerlessness are made even more acute when death comes knocking at our door, and we are forced to face it directly" (Moller 2000). Many of us go through life as if it were never-ending. The hard truth is that we will all get old, we will sicken, and we will all die!

Hanging On

Even with all the advances in plastic surgery, artificial implants, surgical procedures, and medicines, we will get old. Regardless of all the procedures and implants to which you may have subjected yourself, eventually, they will be for naught. So rather than aging gracefully and maintaining a youthful look because of healthy living, we look for quick fixes. My wife often laughs and says that she wants to grow old with grace and dignity, and with soft wrinkles because she earned them.

While we have indeed conquered many illnesses, at least in the Western world, new diseases arise while others are made more virulent through mutations. This will become increasingly prevalent because of modern advances in world travel, along with our constant tampering with nature. So, today, we have AIDS, and quite a few drug-resistant infections such as VRE, MRSA, C-DIFF, and tuberculosis. Include those organisms that humanity has meddled with to create biological weapons, and you can see that we have not conquered anything but have potentially created illnesses that could wipe out a good portion of the planet's human population.

Some of these "superbugs" are the direct result of the indiscriminate use of antibiotics. We have an enormous array of medications, all of which have incredible potential to create other disorders that were not previously present. So, you are given medications. Then, you are given other medications to counteract the adverse effects of the original medication, and on, and on!

And yet, a substantial number of our ailments are self-limiting. A self-limiting illness is one that will resolve itself without lasting effects on the person. Unfortunately, we live in a society that is ruled by the clock, and, as a result, we seek immediate resolutions to all problems. This propels us to seek medical intervention where none is needed.

Regrettably, many physicians respond by treating rather than educating the public for fear of unfavorable reviews. Sadly, we are all led to believe that we can conquer our mortality.

Our instinct of survival is hardwired to guarantee the continuation of the species. I firmly believe that part of this instinctual survival sense includes the formation of binding relationships to the material aspects of our existence. These are illusory anchors that represent the solidity of our material world. Unfortunately, these attachments to loved ones, material things, and the out-of-reach wishes associated with them lead to much pain and suffering.

So, as death approaches, we fight to hang on because of our associations to the physical world and our loved ones. Family and friends that share that same attachment will also cling to the dying one, which results in prolonging the dying process.

To illustrate, a friend of mine started to write an anecdote for this book, and he told me that he could not go on writing. I asked him why and he said, *As I was writing the anecdote associated with my mother's death, I came to the realization that I had put my mother through so much and that it was my fault.* There was also a feeling of guilt because he found it extremely difficult being close to her when she was dying. He felt that he couldn't help her at that time. I know this person well, and I know that he was, in all respects, a loving and caring son. He was one who sacrificed much on behalf of his ailing mother. He is not to blame, for he acted out of love and guidance from his mother's physicians. His natural inclination was not to let go.

It is not unusual for family members to feel remorse at having unnecessarily prolonged their loved one's death. Once again, we recall the old proverb that is packed with meaning: *The road to hell is paved with good intentions*. This proverb was first published in *A Collection of English Probers* (1670) by John Ray (Ray 2019). Simply put, our intentions, however noble they may be, may have very undesirable consequences. We must learn to think, not about ourselves, and what *we* are feeling, but about the one facing the end of life. If you are the one facing the end of your life's journey, then it is about you and what you want.

Another situation in which I was directly involved exemplifies how a dying person may cling to life to fulfill the desire to see a loved one before letting go. I distinctly recall being called by a friend of the family. His father was slowing dying, suffering from advanced dementia and sepsis (infection). My father and I went to spend some time with the family. I knew him well and knew how much he loved his grandchildren. His grandchildren were all close by, except one grandson that was in the military. After spending some time with them, I whispered in his ear that it was okay to go, that his grandson was in another state, and could not arrive fast enough but that he would see him from the other side. The next day I went to work at the hospital when I received a call from my father to tell me that he had passed away early that morning and that he had died peacefully. His beloved grandson arrived in time to bid him farewell. This is but one reason why a dying person may hang on to life.

We must remember that death "…comes in its own time, in its own way." And that it "…is as unique as the individual who is experiencing it" (Karnes 2014). Unfortunately, there are other reasons why the dying may linger past their allotted time on this earth:

- The desire to see someone they love or feel their presence one last time. Remember that the dying will often hang on not for themselves, but for their loved ones.

- Unfinished business. This could be anything from the very materialistic (bonds to money, property, fame, etc.) to repairing a rift among family members.

- Fear of death and what may come after death. This fear can arise regardless of religious beliefs or a lack thereof. I have seen professed atheists ask for forgiveness, "just in case." This is especially powerful if the person fears some sort of afterlife punishment for real or perceived wrongs. Guilt feelings will fuel the fear of death due to the idea of afterlife retribution. One of the many reasons why belief systems are important is that they help to clear-up those guilt feelings.

- Fear for what may happen to those they love after their death. This fear can involve things such as financial concerns, family unity and cohesiveness, and concerns for an already ailing spouse or child.

- Reluctance at relinquishing control to the inevitability of death.

- The enormous pull felt by the dying person from family members that are begging them not to go. This is extremely powerful! Remember that even if the patient is comatose, the spirit can still hear.

During my career, I have offered advice to many families and patients going through this process. I have developed a sense of timing regarding these cases. I do not approach the family unless they are open to the subject for discussion, and only after I have established a good rapport, something that occurs quite frequently. I advise them to speak to their loved one, individually, and in private. "For some it is a time to give and receive forgiveness" (McEntyre 2015). I recommend leaving nothing unsaid, to ask for forgiveness for real or perceived transgressions, and to promise that those left behind will continue to love and look out after each other. Doing this is extremely healing for the dying person, and for family and friends. Unburdening real or perceived transgressions against a loved one can be quite cathartic. You would be surprised at the difference this makes for the dying. Usually, once this occurs, the patient will die soon thereafter and in peace.

Bidding a loved one farewell is perhaps one of the hardest and most compassionate actions that you can perform on behalf of someone you love. "Even if you don't want them to die. Even if you think you can't live without them, … you should let them cross over. And sometimes they need to know it's okay for them to leave. In fact, sometimes they're waiting for your permission to go" (Dyck 2011). Our instinctual response is to hang on to those we love because of the bonds and unrealistic dreams that we have forged. Remember that, in most cases, people know or sense when they have embarked on that final journey. If you outwardly deny the reality of the situation, the person that is dying will often go along with it to spare your feelings.

We should not forget that love is often very possessive and selfish. I know, without a doubt, that most people do not want to lose a loved one regardless of their age. We face the empty room, our memories, our feelings toward our loved one, the smiles, jokes, caresses, and the myriad of things that made us love that very special person! And yet, the true essence of them is the spirit which is manifesting in their physical body. It is that essence, that consciousness, which is undying. We try to come to terms with our transient existence and those we love. We tell ourselves, when it is an older person at death's door, that they have had a full life. We feel the death of a child so much more because of their innocence and the fact that they did not get a chance to experience life. Remember that death does not discriminate; it is the great equalizer.

Regardless of how deep and abiding your love, try not to say to a loved one that is dying, "Please don't leave me," "I don't know what I will do without you," or any similar statement. It is okay to tell them how much you love them and promise to take care of yourself and the rest of the family. The inability of the dying patient to let go may indicate "…unfinished business or the need for a reconciliation that has been previously unidentified" (Williams-Murphy 2011). Give them permission to die by perhaps saying something like, *If it's your time to go, then go; it's okay for you to go, and we'll continue to care for each other*. However deep and abiding your love is, the focus should only be on yourself if you are the one dying. Otherwise, the focus should be on your loved one that is dying and not yourself. Love fully, completely immerse yourself in that love, cherish it, nurture it, but love without unreasonable desires. Love unconditionally by loving the essence, the spirit that is embodied in your loved one, for that is what will never cease. And, when you love to such depths, the greatest act of love is letting go when the time is right.

Letting Go

We form such powerful bonds that "…we are terrified of letting go, in fact, of living at all, since learning to live is learning to let go. And this is the tragedy and the irony of our struggle to hold on: not only is it impossible, but it brings us the very pain we are seeking to avoid" (Rinpoche 2002). Giving a dying person permission to go is NOT wishing their death! It is, indeed, the ultimate act of selfless love! We, the ones left behind, are the ones that will bear the burden of our loss or, better yet, our separation from those we love. Allow your loved one a "good death" by allowing them to die at home, whenever possible, surrounded by familiar faces instead of strangers.

I have witnessed countless deaths in the intensive care unit, many of which occurred while the patient was alone. In some cases, they were alert, and in others, they were not. Remember, however, that hearing is the last sense that is lost. Think of the peace and enormous sense of love that your loved one will experience while you are holding their hand, and while you are telling them how much you love them and that it is okay to die! Letting go of a loved one or holding on to them is an intimate and very personal act.

I often feel that when we mourn the death of someone we love, we are mourning our loss rather than their death. Why do I say this? Because, even though we know that our loved one will no longer be in pain, and they will no longer be suffering a lingering and often painful death, we, on the other hand, are the ones that are left behind. We mourn for that which we had and enjoyed but can no longer have in this life. We cry for the things that we no longer have, and we keenly feel the pain of losing that attachment. We also mourn the emptiness of unfulfilled aspirations: the plans for the future, the laughter, the joy, the love, the very presence of the one that is gone from this world. It is not uncommon for the dying to offer the living relief. Remember, the bonds of love are not so easily broken!

Letting go of your attachments and their associated expectations require that you take a close and intimate look at your true self. You must bare your soul and subject it to scrutiny. There are certain basic aspects of your being that you need to look at under the light of truth. These same aspects can be applied to a loved one that is dying:

- First, ask yourself what makes your life worth living? Based on your knowledge of self, or that of a loved one, would you want to go on, or would they want to go on under these conditions? If you can, look back into your life and then move forward to the present. Do this because, as you should realize by now, everything changes. What were the things that you enjoyed the most? Was it your independence, your creativity, your ability to interact with family and friends? Was it the work you did with your own hands, the things you created, the music you played and enjoyed, dancing with your partner, playing catch with your son or daughter? I know that as we age, there will be activities that we can no longer perform or enjoy. But it is ultimately your independence and ability to interact, in some meaningful fashion, that matters. Think about these things and then assess your current abilities to continue those interactions. Think about those things that would make life not worth living. Think about whether you want to go on in your current condition or not.

- Next, you should look at those things that you would not want to endure, such as the things that would rob you of your quality of life. These will vary from person to person, but I will share with you those things that would make my life not worth living: I like to be independent and able to look after my own needs; being bedridden and unable to wipe my own rear-end is not something that I would like; I would find it very difficult to contemplate a feeding tube or a colostomy bag; nor would I like becoming a burden to my loving wife, even though I know she would care for me until my last breath. Not wanting to live under certain conditions is NOT a sign of weakness or of being cowardly. Remember the following: You do NOT have to suffer to atone for real or perceived past transgressions. What happens in the afterlife depends on how you depart from this material plane. It is an intimate dialogue between you and your Maker. Make peace with yourself and the world around you. Repentance occurs in the heart and the spirit. Words of contrition are meaningless if they do not come from the depths of your heart and soul. Look forward to a new life without pain and suffering and take solace in the fact that you WILL see your loved ones again!

- Consider what it would be like to die in an intensive care unit while enduring techno-hell. It has been called techno-hell for a reason, for it is that very same medical technology that can prolong your life that will also prolong your dying. Is going to a nursing home or an LTAC an option for you? The truth is that you would find it difficult to meet a healthcare worker that would willingly go to a nursing home or an LTAC. They are not all the same, but the good ones are financially beyond the reach of most people. I do not know about you, but I would opt to go home.

- Would you be willing to be kept alive if your ability to think and communicate was gone? I accept it as true that the brain is the mechanism that allows the lifeforce to express itself in our material plane of existence. Once the brain is damaged, that spirit can no longer express itself, and it is left in a state of limbo, not fully attached and not totally freed. If you find yourself hanging on or wishing that a loved one would hang on, try to find out the reasons why. Is it for your family or yourself? What is the purpose of hanging on? What will it solve? Family members may not want you to go, but if it is your time, then go in peace. They have their own paths to follow as you have followed yours.

- What happens to the material things that you leave behind should be of no consequence to you. You may have heard the old saying, "You can't take it with you." Well, it is true. Being concerned with the material aspects of life during the dying process is a sign of being seriously attached to the material world. It is understandable for you to worry about the material aspects of those that are left behind. It is acceptable for you to try and provide for those you love, even after your death. In the end, however, each individual has his or her own karmic path and spiritual evolution, which includes their trials and tribulations in the material plane. This is not a cop-out or an excuse to not care. It is a reality, for, regardless of what you do, your private script will take its course.

- Realize that some situations may seem hopeless, so I would suggest that you give things a chance to play out. I do not wish for death since I thoroughly enjoy my life. Thus, I would give thought to various possibilities, which, of course, would vary from case to case. This is one of the many reasons why having the truth is so important. It will give you the freedom to make intelligent decisions regarding your future.

With a true prognosis, I will be able to make the correct decisions and preparations for my death. It will give me a chance to live the rest of my days in the best possible way that I desire and not to be surrounded by strangers, machines, tubes, medications, and so on! I prefer to die at home, surrounded by the love of my family and the company of my friend, my lover, my partner, my Twin Flame—my wife! I welcome hospice care (they are truly wonderful and caring individuals), and I will accept the medications to relieve pain. I want to make my transition from this plane of existence to the next while conscious. After all, that will be the beginning of another great adventure! I do not wish to be resuscitated or have heroic measures performed if I am dying.

The process of dying does not necessarily involve a terminal illness or condition. Ultimately, our lifeforce will start to diminish, and we will enter that last phase. I would not want to be intubated or put on life support if there is no chance of regaining a meaningful existence. I trust my wife implicitly, and I know that she will honor my wishes as I will honor hers. I do not want to waste precious moments in doctor's offices, emergency rooms, unnecessary hospitalizations, futile procedures, etc. I would rather spend that time with my loved one, in the present, in the here-and-now!

The very same thoughts expressed above can be applied if you are facing the death of a loved one. First, obtain the truth, for, without it, you will be powerless. It is okay to grieve prior to losing a loved one. This is called *anticipatory grief*. It is experienced before the actual loss of a loved one, based on the knowledge that the person is indeed dying.

Focus on the Positive

Try not to shed your tears in the presence of the loved one that is dying. Why? Because this can easily prolong the dying process since your loved one will, in most cases, want to avoid hurting you. However, if you do cry in their presence, do not feel guilty, but rather than dwell on the negative aspects of the situation, try to focus on the positive. Think not of death and dying but of the fact that life continues beyond physical death. Focus on all the positive and happy occasions of your relationship with the person that is dying. Be grateful for the time that you have spent together. Be grateful for the lessons that you taught each other, the lessons that allowed you to grow as a human being, and the wisdom that was learned through your interactions. Let them know how much they meant to you and that they will be missed. But, above all, give them permission to go and reassure them that you will take care of yourself and that the family will look out for each other. If you believe in an afterlife, then take solace in the fact that death is but an interruption and that, soon, your paths will once again cross.

CB EO

The best and safest thing is to keep a balance in your life, acknowledge the great powers around us and in us. If you can do that, and live that way, you are really a wise man.

Euripides

C３ ８０

Go confidently in the direction of your dreams!
Live the life you've imagined.
As you simplify your life, the laws of the universe will
be simpler.

Henry David Thoreau

CHAPTER SIX

Putting it All Together

❖

To Those in The Healthcare Fields

We, as healthcare providers, should always have one thing and one thing only on our minds, and that is our patients. I hope that everyone in health care, including doctors, nurses, respiratory therapists, physician's assistants, nurse practitioners, and anyone else that encounters patients and their families, will have had some degree of exposure to the content matter of this book.

Regardless of how our medical education has indoctrinated us, the truth remains that death and dying is a reality that we must address. Furthering one's education on behalf of our patients and their families should continually be pursued. In health care, the subject matter of death and dying is usually relegated to the back. It is often treated as an afterthought. As a result, we may find ourselves at odds when confronting death and dying.

There is this fear of reaching out to the family or patient. It is indeed a sensitive topic, but one that will not disappear. It is the responsibility of our education system to incorporate the materials needed to address these issues as we care for our patients and their families.

Remember Why You Chose Your Profession

Hopefully, you chose your profession because you had a deep and abiding desire to help other human beings. If you chose health care as a profession for some other reason, you are still responsible for carrying out your duties to the best of your abilities. Otherwise, it is time to consider another profession. I make these statements because I have come across healthcare practitioners that chose their profession because it pays well and because of job security. In other cases, it was because it was expected of them. If you find that this profession is not for you, then do yourself, your patients, and their families a favor and find a different one.

Remember to treat your patients as if they were family members. Keep in mind the old Biblical proverb, *Do unto others as you would have them do unto you.* How would you or someone you love like to be treated? In any event, the best healthcare practitioners that I have ever met in my lengthy career chose this profession because they felt that it was their calling, a vocation.

There is a Difference Between Being a Practitioner of Your Profession and a Healer

Our biomedical model of medicine treats human beings as a malfunctioning organism that requires technological interventions to restore it to a functioning or semi-functioning level. When you approach your profession from the biomedical perspective, you are simply a practitioner, however good you may be. Unfortunately, we compartmentalize all things, including our professions. When this occurs, we become so focused on the physical that we miss a multitude of things that occur on the mental, emotional, and spiritual levels—that together comprise a healthy state.

I use the term healer in a quasi-traditional fashion. A healer is an individual that recognizes that people are so much more than a complex biological organism. A healer will consider the multidimensional reality of all human beings, that is, the physical, mental, emotional, and spiritual. A healer recognizes that when one of these is ailing, the other three are also affected. Therefore, we should all be sensitive to the individual as a whole. This does not mean that we all should become psychiatrists, psychologists, or spiritual counselors. However, being aware and sensitive will bring to light problems that were previously unknown, and that could be impacting the health and recovery of your patient. This requires a deeper level of communication. All it takes is a few extra moments to observe, truly listen, and *feel* the energy or atmosphere surrounding your patient, and anyone else that may be present.

Human beings are also social creatures, and we thrive on human touch and interaction. The loss of such interactions could potentially lead to the syndrome known as *Failure to Thrive*. Failure to Thrive "…is not a single disease or medical condition; rather, it's a nonspecific manifestation of an underlying physical, mental, or psychosocial condition" and there are three precipitating factors among others that can lead to this condition: "Depression," "Desertion by family, friends (social isolation)," and "Despair (giving up)" (Ali 2015). I believe that this process may start when an individual senses that their journey in this lifetime is coming to an end. More so when they feel or intuit that others simply do not care or, in some cases, because a distancing has occurred between the person and other members of the family. It is as if these individuals have lost their will to live! I have also seen individuals begin to withdraw from social interactions as they prepare themselves for what lies ahead.

Being aware of the multidimensional aspects of human beings could bring to light subtle issues that may otherwise escape you. This insight into your patient will allow you to seek the appropriate assistance.

Communication Goes Beyond Mere Words

Communication occurs through words, facial expressions, body postures, eye contact, and, yes, at the energy level. I know that we are all harassed by time constraints and the fact that "big brother" is always watching. We have enormous workloads, hundreds of medications to give, charting, calls to take, and a myriad of other duties. Everyone is in a hurry, and when this happens, we begin to lose touch with our patients and their family members. To top it off, we have our personal lives and whatever problems that may entail.

Know that a lack of communication is one of the most frequent complaints from patients and family members, especially regarding the doctors involved in the case. I understand the pressures that physicians experience, especially with the tremendous number of patients that they may see. Nonetheless, a few extra minutes will do wonders for their practice and, more importantly, for their patients.

The fact remains, however, that we are there for our patients and for no other reason! Forget the scripted verbiage that we are told to use. Most patients have a built-in lie-detecting radar, and they can tell the difference. Be genuine in your concern; do not fake it!

When talking to your patients, treat them as human beings. Treat them as you would in a regular social situation and not with a stiff neck, deadpan approach, which can translate to cold, distant, and uncaring. Develop a *feel* for your patients.

For example, there are many patients that I talk to using their first name while others I use the more formal Mr., Ms., or Mrs. Others I greet as *Hey, how's it going today?* In many cases, I joke with them and make them laugh. I still teach them, give them their medications, and provide reassurances whenever possible. I answer their medical questions as I teach them, and for those things beyond my scope, I refer them to the right individuals. Use your intuition and your knowledge, but above all, be real!

With patients that are in distress, I use a hands-on approach such as placing my hand on their shoulder or their hand. I also use what I call a *healing voice*. Words and the way that they are used can and do have a powerful impact on people. Thus, I modulate my voice so that it carries a sense of peace and tranquility, a voice that speaks of ease and healing. It is a voice that soothes the energy and one that is filled with confidence. This voice, however, is not something that is rehearsed. It is a voice that comes from a sincere desire to soothe those that are ailing. You can fake this voice, but the effects will not be the same. Is it always successful? No, for it depends on the patient's receptivity. In my experience, however, the use of a healing voice will usually have some positive effect/s.

Another way to open the avenue of good communication is by learning how to pronounce someone's name. I do this all the time, and you would be surprised at the positive responses from the patient and others that may be present. There is so much that is vested in a name, including the meaning or significance of that name, ties to ancestry, and the fact that it is intimately intertwined with the person as a whole. Learning to pronounce someone's name is a sign of utmost respect. They now see you as an intelligent and respectful individual.

Cultural and Ethnic Sensitivity

I smile when I take the mandated cultural sensitivity classes. I smile because they are so inadequate and superficial. If you truly want to learn about another culture, then take the time to investigate. Google it! Better yet, ask a member of that culture or get to know someone from that culture. Open your mind and learn. You may be surprised at the wonderful experiences you have been missing.

Moreover, you may be pleasantly surprised at how much we share with other cultures. Focus on the similarities or parallels rather than the differences. One of the best ways of showing cultural sensitivity is by being respectful yet inquisitive.

I often hear co-workers make derogatory comments about other cultures such as, *oh my God, those Spanish people are so loud, and there's a roomful of them!* What you should keep in mind is that your patient has an enormous support network of loving individuals that come in to make that patient feel good. Yes, it is fine to remind them that they are in a hospital but do not belittle these interactions.

Another way of showing cultural sensitivity is by accepting the fact that we live in a multicultural society. Do not be offended when someone is speaking their native language! You would do the same if the situation were reversed. It is natural for people to revert to their native language. Stop being so paranoid as to think that they are talking about you. Do you feel so insecure or self-centered as to think that everyone around you is talking about you? You talk about other people as well, except that you do it behind their backs or behind closed doors. So, who cares what people are saying about you if that is indeed the case! For all you know, they may be praising you.

Be sensitive by accepting the fact that not everyone is able to learn English. English is not an easy language to learn and becomes even more difficult with age. In some cultures, it is not unusual for a homemaker and mother to remain at home caring for the children while the men go out and earn a living. In such cases, the need to acquire the language is not pressing.

There are many reasons why some people do not pick up a language. However, it is not due to disrespect! Should anyone able to learn the language do so? Absolutely! But do not hold it against the elders of any culture. Have compassion and understanding. Walk in their shoes and imagine yourself torn away from your roots, your country, and everything that you have ever known, and imagine being thrust into a foreign society.

Sensitivity and Privacy—a Modern-Day Illusion

Remember that your patients are in an extremely vulnerable position. When they enter a hospital, they are stripped of their independence. They are asked to forgo their rights and entrust their life into the hands of strangers.

George Orwell wrote a dystopian novel called *Nineteen Eighty-Four* (often seen written as *1984*) in which he warned that *Big Brother* was constantly watching (a poster that appeared throughout the world of Oceania). This novel involved a totalitarian government that violated the privacy of its citizens. And, like so many science fiction novels, it is, to a large degree, coming true.

To illustrate, it is a frequent practice today to place cameras in patients' rooms! This is done under the pretext of *safety*. While there is an element of truth regarding patient safety, there is also an underlying factor and a powerful motivating force. Surveillance is used to lower facility costs by decreasing the number of employees required to keep an eye on the patient population. Keep in mind that this is a violation of your privacy.

When admitted to a hospital, you should ask if there is a camera in your room. Look around your room carefully, and if there is one, it is your legal right to refuse being watched. It is a matter of privacy! If you do not do this, then someone may constantly be watching you or someone you love. This is a violation of HIPPA Law! I have witnessed many occasions where a patient had inadvertently exposed himself or herself!

There are certain instances when the use of a camera is acceptable such as in the case of patients that are in danger due to their confused state of mind, dementia, those with suicidal ideation, or suspected drug users.

Being hospitalized leaves one feeling vulnerable and often scared. You are away from the familiar, from your home and loved ones. This situation worsens depending on the acuity or seriousness of the illness. This vulnerability can put people on edge. I have taken care of many nursing home patients that you can tell were not treated properly. They recoil at the slightest touch, and you can see the fear in their eyes! The same thing is often evidenced in individuals in abusive relationships. We need to be careful not to transfer our own issues to those that we care for on a day-to-day basis.

Be Genuine and Never Assume

Do not lie to your patients. Be honest and forthcoming with them. They deserve your respect. Do not assume that your patient is ignorant regarding medical issues. Even if they are, never assume that they are incapable of understanding.

I often hear co-workers complain about the patient or family member that is always asking questions. To me, that is a sign of intelligence and of an individual that is in touch with what is going on in their lives or that of someone they love. Not everyone is litigious! Let them know that it is okay to ask questions. I encourage my patients to question, for knowledge gives power and security.

You would be surprised at the number of times that a family member or a patient has caught an error in medications! Also, you may not know your patient's background and education. I have taken care of patients from all levels of society: doctors, nurses, politicians, nuns, priests, police officers, lawyers, respiratory therapists, CEOs of hospitals, teachers, professors, writers, gang members, prostitutes, and one of the last Mafia bosses in Tampa, Florida.

In other words, you will never know, so treat your patients with respect. Never forget the built-in *lie detector*. You would be surprised at the number of people that let me know when someone is not genuine because they can feel it and see it.

Also, healthcare institutions do not want you to tell the truth regarding things such as staff-to-patient ratios, as well as other practices aimed at increasing admissions.

I know that the establishments want you to remain quiet about certain things. The best policy is to be honest. The quickest way to end up with bad reviews or a lawsuit is to lie to the patient and family.

In fact, one study that was conducted over a decade ago showed that "… patients are less likely to sue, even where there was negligence, as long as the physician told them of the mistake and told the truth" (L'Hommedieu Stankus 2009). I find that most people are quite understanding and accommodating when treated with respect.

A few years ago, I took my wife to the emergency room due to lower abdominal pain. After extensive testing, she was diagnosed with a "mild and uncomplicated diverticulitis." The emergency department (ED) physician wanted to admit her to have an invasive endoscopy. She refused admission because we knew what steps to take to minimize or prevent future flare-ups. The next day I found out, through a friend of mine who is a case manager, that my wife had been labeled as a "missed admission."

Unfortunately, there are times when I am not able to go back and take one of my patients off their treatment in a timely manner, but I apologize while being honest. If I am occupied with another patient, I let them know that it was not a matter of forgetfulness.

The Difficult Patient

Yes, they do exist! And it has become worse in this day and age, where patients are treated as customers instead of patients. People go into hospitals today, thinking that they are going to be staying in some fancy hotel. The fault lies squarely with the system that is concerned with the bottom line.

Indeed, there are and always will be those individuals that try our patience, understanding, and compassion. They make it a point to be obnoxious, demanding, insulting, denigrating, and confrontational. You should not have to be subjected to that abuse! I know that it is difficult to feel compassionate toward people like that but try to remain as understanding and sympathetic as you can since their problems go beyond the physical.

These individuals are also sick in other ways that may not be so overt. If you become negative, then the situation will only deteriorate, for like attracts like. Try to remain positive and calm as long as you can, and when you feel that you cannot, walk away whenever possible. I have seen individuals such as these turn around and change because of being bombarded with positive energy from their caregivers! Was it easy? No, it was not!

Final Thoughts

A great many of us walk through life without pausing to consider the deeper aspects of our existence. We live in an extremely demanding society, one that is ruled by a timetable. Living has to do with enjoying your life and those that you love. Do not postpone that enjoyment! I am not advocating irresponsible behaviors of any type, for we must work and earn a living to support our families. Unfortunately, a great many people tend to focus on the material aspects of living only to discover that life has passed them by and, by then, it may be too late.

I remember many years ago, taking care of an individual in his early thirties, married with two small sons. He was a hard-working man with his own business. This patient came in with a major heart attack. He survived the cardiac event, but his heart function was so poor that the doctor told him not to do any strenuous work because his heart could not meet the demands. His entire focus had been to make his business successful to support his family. In the end, however, neither one materialized. The physician informed the patient that his heart attack was due to several factors, including the tremendous stress that he was experiencing from his business.

Strive to become self-aware and learn to live in the present. Enjoy each moment with your loved ones. We are undoubtedly creatures of habit. We establish routines to such an extent that a substantial number of hours go by, and tasks are performed with little conscious thought. We even tend to drive to and from work on "auto-pilot." We also tend to take things for granted until reality knocks on our door.

Never leave home angry or without gently kissing your spouse, and your children if you are a parent. Do not waste precious time in meaningless squabbles with your loved ones. Do not let selfishness rule your life. Instead, be giving and forgiving. Practice compassion, understanding, acceptance, tolerance, and try to rise above. Our lives run on a clock. This clock is winding down all the time, and the process begins at birth! No, this is not a fatalistic point of view but a reality check.

The fact that you have been reading this book tells me that you are interested in expanding your propriospect or worldview and, in so doing, preparing for the future so that you can truly live. Read and re-read this book, take notes, read further, investigate and, most importantly, think! In preparing for the nonmanipulable aspects of our existence, you will begin to experience life more fully.

By living in the here-and-now, you will become aware of the true wonders that surround us, and you will gain peace and a degree of wisdom. You will experience life from a whole new perspective. What you take out of this book and how much you apply to your life is, of course, up to you. Your decisions will affect you and those you love and cherish. We walk through life holding

Death's hand, but we are so accustomed to this that we have lost that awareness.

We are all familiar with Charles Dickens' *A Christmas Carol*. The final visitation is that of the Grim Reaper or Death, a reminder that time passes relentlessly and that we are indeed mortal. After going through a review of his life and the realization of his own possible demise, Ebenezer Scrooge changes and truly begins to enjoy life! But this change comes about after the realization that he was missing out on life. He finally realized all the things that could have been! One way to interpret this classic is that it is never too late to change, that we should live each day with awareness and enjoy life.

Regardless of how healthy you are, how well you eat, how much you exercise, your human frailty will catch up. Continue to take care of yourself so that you may enjoy your life to the fullest. Do not take life for granted in the process, for it is a precious gift that will eventually end.

To prepare for this eventuality is an act of love for yourself and for those you love. Do not live in fear of what may be, for the future is determined by every step you take in the present. Think about the issues surrounding this topic, discuss them with your family, and then make plans. These plans can always be changed should you change your mind. It is in everyone's best interest to have your wishes and plans made known to those that you love.

You may be in the best of health now, but, as I have mentioned before, change is the only constant in this universe. I have seen healthy and strong individuals succumb to an unexpected set of events such as a devastating infection, a drug interaction, a surgical procedure, or an accident, to name a few. I am by no means suggesting that you live in abject fear filled with morbid thoughts of impending doom, for life is too precious to waste away with such considerations. Take a realistic view of your life or that of a loved one.

Things to Consider

The most difficult part will probably be bringing up the subject, since most people avoid such topics. Whether you are thinking of yourself or someone that you love, the process is the same for anyone regardless of age. What follows is a list of suggestions for you to consider when making any decision regarding one's death or that of a loved one. Feel free to modify or add to this list. Write things down, legalize when appropriate, and have a conversation about this subject with those you trust.

- First and foremost, carefully consider the quality of life. This is quite subjective and will vary from person to person. It is up to you to determine what you would consider good quality in life. This is extremely important when making end-of-life decisions. If you or a loved one is facing a devastating condition and prognosis, make sure to assess the factors related to the quality of your life. Pay attention to those that you love. What drives them? What aspects of life did they cherish the most? Debate these issues with those that are close to you. Know your loved ones and be aware of what they would consider a good quality of life. Would you consider being in a consistent vegetative state or being confined to a bed and unable to move, talk, or take care of your bodily functions a good quality of life? Is being mentally aware of all things that occur around you while confined to a bed and being unable to interact with the world around you acceptable? Think in terms of maintaining your autonomy or that of a loved one. Make your own decisions or allow someone you love to make them, then honor those decisions. This is one very important issue to consider when determining what you would or would not accept for yourself. This is an extremely significant topic to chat about with loved ones, that is, what they or you would consider acceptable or not!

- When considering the above, think of any comorbidity factors that you or a loved one may have: advanced or uncontrolled diabetes, kidney insufficiency, kidney failure, advanced COPD, cancer, liver failure, dementia, HIV, and chronic cardiac issues to name a few. Think of the impact such conditions would have at the end of life.

- Pay attention to your intuition. What is your body telling you? Do not ignore the signals it provides. Your body communicates with you in many ways. Learn to listen to what it is telling you because listening to these signals can make a huge difference in the outcome of many illnesses. There is a *knowing* associated with the process of death and dying. Listen to your body and listen to what loved ones say regarding this matter, even if there is a reluctance to examine these issues openly.

- If you choose to fight for your life, regardless of the odds, then do so with intelligence and passion. The worst thing that you can do is fight half-heartedly. You must strive to maintain a positive frame of mind amid the chaos. Depression and anxiety, when prolonged, will adversely affect your immune system (your immune system is of primary importance in fighting cancer and other diseases). I would investigate all healing modalities, both mainstream and alternative. Be thorough and unbiased in your research. This is the time to open your mind to all possibilities. Consider the healing properties of food and plants. Naturally, if you start taking alternative medicines, check with your physician. Keep in mind that there are excellent reference books on the interactions between pharmaceuticals and herbal preparations. Do not allow negative individuals into your life. Instead, surround yourself, if possible, with people that are positive. Learn methods of meditation and visualization. Prayers are also very powerful. You will either win or lose this fight and, in the end, you will know when it is time to stop fighting. The decision is yours alone.

- Arm yourself with knowledge. Base your decisions on facts, not wishes. But do not disregard your intuition, for it comes from a much higher place. We can all fool ourselves or those we love through wishful thinking and the inability to face the facts that are in front of you. Your intuition is precious; therefore, pay attention, since it could save your life. Pay attention to your intuitive self and learn to discern true intuition from self-generated thoughts and ideas.

- Strive to avoid unreasonable attachments for they will inevitably lead to much suffering both in this life and the next. We often hurt those that we love the most, or we are hurt by those that love us the most but not necessarily because of any malicious intent. Will your decisions be based on the best interests of yourself or that of a loved one, or based on desires and unreasonable attachments? Remember that we grieve for our loss and how it affects us; those that are gone are in a better place. What someone else thinks you should or should not do in the end may not be in your best interest. Do not hold back those that you profess to love because that is an act of selfishness. Unconditional love entails the ability to let go. Let yourself go when it is time. Life does not end after we leave this plane of existence. Let go of unreasonable attachments. Love the spirit, not only the physical but take care of the physical for it is the vehicle through which the spirit manifests in this world. It is the spirit that lives on, and it is within the spirit that the bonds of love are carried.

- Assess and carefully reassess your health status. You can then change your living will, if desired, to reflect changing conditions and opinions.

- The course of a disease/prognosis is beyond the power of the healthcare team. They are NOT infallible! All they can do is give you their professional opinion, which is based on their knowledge, experience, and individualized view of the world. Do not blame them for the vagaries of life because all things change. Be grateful for their kind care, their compassion, knowledge, and expertise.

- Carefully consider all the possible outcomes of accepting heroic measures at the end of life. Will you be prolonging your life or prolonging your death? Remember that palliative chemotherapy and radiation therapy are designed to extend the inevitability of your death for X amount of time. In such cases, you need to know that a) the outcome is inevitable, and b) that the extra time may be miserable as a result of the side effects of these treatment regimens. Keep in mind that palliative care, while possibly extending your life, many also exacerbate your suffering. The question to ask yourself and your loved ones is simple: *Will the final outcome change?* If you are willing to undertake procedures that will prolong your suffering or that of someone you love, then try to answer the following question: What is the purpose behind my decision?

- You have the right to request or demand, if necessary, a realistic prognosis, and realistic outcomes of suggested interventions, but do this in a holistic fashion. Look at things from all angles so that you will be able to make an informed decision. Do not be misled by false promises. It is your legal right to know the truth! But remember that the only constant in this universe is that everything changes.

- You are entitled to rely on physicians to tell you what you need to know about the condition of your body. You have the right to chart your own destiny, and the physicians involved must supply you with the unbiased facts that you need.

- It is your legal right to refuse all medical treatments or procedures if you are mentally competent. Should your mental competency be questioned, your durable power of attorney or your healthcare surrogate will step in to ensure that your last wishes will be honored.

Things to Do

- Advance directives. A surrogate healthcare designation and a living will are of tremendous importance. Make sure to include a DNR and a DNI clause within your living will (or as separate documents) if that is your wish. Be sure to include a HIPAA (Health Insurance Portability and Accountability Act of 1996) document so that your healthcare proxy can have access to your medical records. Also, include what you would or would not accept, such as mechanical ventilation, chemical life support (drugs), feeding tubes, dialysis, chemotherapy, radiation therapy, surgery, etc. Make sure that all documents are legally binding but keep in mind that notarizing a document does not mean that it is legally binding! These documents should be prepared by an attorney for your own protection. Remember that laws vary according to the state of residence, so be sure to check your state laws and requirements.

- If possible, obtain a DPOA and carefully choose a person that will carry out your last wishes. This individual is legally assigned to make healthcare decisions on your behalf, which are based on your wishes or the wishes of the person involved. Carefully inform yourself on your state's DPOA laws to avoid future headaches.

- Make your medical wishes known to your family, close friends, and your doctor. Provide copies of documents if necessary. You will know when it is time to create the legal documentation mentioned above but, in the meantime, make sure that you let other members of the family know what your wishes are and write them down (dated and signed).

- I know that this is a difficult topic to discuss. Therefore, think of ways in which you can start such a conversation. For example, Laura Grimme McCullough, R.N., A.C.M. suggested the following: *I would like to discuss my final wishes, including my funeral arrangements. What would be a good time?* Or, *Mom, Dad, as you know, I have laid out my end-of-life wishes. I would like to go over yours in order to make sure that I carry out your wishes.* Some people will welcome the discussion while others will shy away from such topics. Do not be angry or disappointed. Respect their wishes and let them know that you are willing to discuss these issues at any point in time.

- Create a medical portfolio that includes legal copies of your healthcare documents and health information (including major illnesses that are chronic in nature, and previous major surgeries). Create a complete list of all medications: name, dosage, and frequency, and carry a copy in your wallet or purse at all times. If handwritten, be sure that it is legible. This list can also be created in computer programs such as Word, Excel, PDF, or even your email program. Keep it updated. If you do not know how to do this or you are unable, have someone you trust do it for you. Provide copies of your medical portfolio to your healthcare surrogate, and/or DPOA, and trusted family members. Keep this portfolio where it can be easily accessed in case of an emergency. Try to make sure that, if you must go to the emergency department, you or someone you trust brings your health portfolio. This will help the healthcare team to honor your wishes and provide you with adequate care based on your wishes. It will also help to avoid possible medical errors involving medications. Be thorough with your information! You would be amazed at the number of patients that provide incomplete information to physicians and nurses. This is crucial, especially in an emergency.

- If you or a loved one is diagnosed with a life-threatening condition or chronic illness that is progressive in nature, then create a list of questions to ask your physicians and other healthcare professionals. Make sure to include the following questions:

1. Ask what the diagnosis is, for clarity.

2. Ask for the truth about the prognosis.

3. If extensive tests or treatments are being discussed, then ask the reasons why they are needed.

4. If they want you to undergo treatment, then ask what impact it will have (if any) on the final outcome and any and all possible side effects.

5. Ask if any of the offered interventions will change the final outcome.

6. Ask if a treatment being offered is curative or merely palliative in nature.

7. Ask if any of the treatments offered will impact your quality of life

8. Ask and learn about hospice care

9. Ask about pain management options.

- Think carefully regarding burial, embalming, cremation, etc. The funeral industry is there to sell you the best package. They may be sincere or sound sincere, but nonetheless, it is a business. Make these decisions ahead of time, and, in doing so, you will alleviate your loved ones from having to make them.

These issues can be discussed regardless of your age or current health status. In the case of children, it is the parent's responsibility to think of the proper steps to take. I am aware of how difficult this would be, since no parent wants to contemplate the death of a child. However, the fact remains that it does indeed occur. Once you have discussed and arrived at some decision regarding these end-of-life issues, then go on with the business of living. As time passes, you may want to revisit the documents to see if there is anything that should be changed. Except that this time, you should strive to do so with awareness! Leave a legacy of love, compassion, understanding, kindness, and, whenever possible, altruism.

Final Words

End-of-life issues are quite extensive, and, for that reason, I have covered the mental, emotional, and spiritual aspects of this topic in my second book, *Now That I Am Dead: What I Should Know at the End of Life*. In the meantime, I want to leave you with the following thoughts:

- In accepting our finitude, we truly begin to live! The recognition and acceptance that our physical existence is finite will then focus our attention on life as it is unfolding before our very eyes.

- Life does NOT end with the death of the physical body! It is merely a transition from one state of existence to another. We are all interconnected, for we cannot exist outside of that energy field. Yes, we are outwardly different and, yet, there are more similarities than differences. It is how you focus your perception that matters in the end.

- All living organisms on this planet have a finite physical existence, but our consciousness does not perish with the death of the body. Our spirit continues to exist, carrying with it the experiences of each lifetime.

- Do not fear death, for it is merely a rite of passage. The spirit and consciousness continue after the death of the physical. We must enjoy every moment with those that we love and cherish every moment of our journey in this lifetime.

Our finitude should entrench us in living with a heightened awareness and, in so doing, our lives will have the most beautiful ripple-effect upon the lives of others! Finally, questions will arise that are more difficult to answer. These questions deal with existential issues, such as has your life had any purpose, meaning, or value? If you are a religious person, you may wonder if it is God's will that you suffer or if suffering is part of your karma. Karma (at its most basic) refers to the force exerted by your actions that will influence the quality of your present life or future incarnations. Simplistically stated, "What comes around, goes around." Believers and nonbelievers may be concerned with the idea as to whether or not they have left some positive legacy. Others may be concerned about what their church members will think about them and their decision. Most importantly, you may question your decision and wonder if you are *playing God*.

ᑫ ᒍ

Cʒ ৪৩

Suggested Reading

Callanan, Maggie and Patricia Kelley. Final Gifts: Understanding the Special Awareness, Needs, and Communications of the Dying. (New York: Simon & Schuster Paperbacks, 1992).

Gawande, Atul, M.D. Being Mortal. (New York: Metropolitan Books, 2014).

Harris, Trudy, R.N. Glimpses of Heaven: True Stories of Hope & Peace at the End of Life's Journey. (Grand Rapids, MI.: Revell, 2008).

Kübler-Ross, Elisabeth, M.D. Death: The Final Stage of Growth. (New York: Touchstone, 1986).

Kübler -Ross, Elisabeth, M.D. On Death & Dying: What the Dying Have to Teach Doctors, Nurses, Clergy & Their Own Families. (New York: Scribner, 1969).

Kübler -Ross, Elisabeth, M.D. On Children and Death: How children and their parents can and do cope with death. (New York: Touchstone, 1983).

Williams-Murphy, Monica, M.D. It's OK To Die. (Place of Publication Not Identified: MKN, LLC, 2011).

Schlitz, Marilyn, PhD. Death Makes Life Possible: Revolutionary Insights on Living, Dying, and the Continuation of Consciousness. (Boulder, CO.: Sounds True, Inc., 2015).

Volandes, Angelo E., M.D. The Conversation: A Revolutionary Plan For End-Of-Life Care. (New York: Bloomsbury Publishing Plc, 2015).

Dunn, Hank. Hard Choices for Loving People: CPR, Feeding Tubes, Comfort Measures, and the Patient with a Serious Illness. (Naples, Florida.: Quality of Life Publishing Co., 2016).

Singh, Kathleen Dowling. The Grace in Dying: A Message of Hope, Comfort, and Spiritual Transformation. (New York, New York: Harper Collins, 2000).

Moller, David Wendell. Life's End: Technocratic Dying in an Age of Spiritual Yearning. (Amityville, New York: Baywood Publishing Co., Inc.).

Karnes, Barbara, R.N., A Time to Live: Living with a Life-Threatening Illness. (Vancouver, WA., Barbara Karnes Books, Inc., 2014).

My Friend, I Care: The Grief Experience. (Vancouver, WA., Barbara Karnes Books, Inc., 2014).

The Eleventh Hour: A caring guide for the hours to minutes before death. (Vancouver, WA., Barbara Karnes Books, Inc., 2014).

Gone From My Sight: The Dying Experience. Vancouver, WA., Barbara Karnes Books, Inc., 2014).

Nuland, Sherwin B, How We Die: Reflections on Life's Final Chapter. (New York, New York. First Vintage Books Edition, January 1995).

Kaufman, Sharon R. …and a time to die: How American Hospitals Shape the End of Life. (Chicago, Illinois. The University of Chicago Press. 2005).

Fitzpatrick, Jeanne, M.D. and Eileen M. Fitzpatrick, J.D. A Better Way of Dying: How to Make

The Best Choices at the End of Life. (New York, New York. Penguin Books Ltd.).

Dan Krauss. Extremis. (Documentary on End-of-Life. 24 minutes. Netflix – Streaming).

Time of Death – Season1. (Documentary - Six Episodes. Amazon Prime). "…an unflinching, intimate look at remarkable people facing their own mortality. Cameras follow these brave, terminally ill individuals as they live out the end of their lives, supported by family, friends, and…"

Randy Bacon and Shannon Bacon. The Last Days of Extraordinary Lives. (Documentary 2010. 86 minutes. Amazon Prime). "In this inspiring and captivating documentary, ordinary people face their last days and yet tell extraordinary stories about their lives and the beautiful experience of living."

Kirby Dick. The End. (Documentary 2004. 84 minutes. Amazon Prime). "One of the most Powerfully intimate films ever made about the final stages of life. The End is a profound and moving chronicle of five hospice patients whose stories are in turns honest, humorous, and heartbreaking."

Death: A Series About Life. (5 episodes. 53 minutes each. Amazon Prime). "We are all going to Die – sooner or later – but there can be great differences in how we relate to death."

৩ ৪০

References

Alfonsi, Sharyn. 2009. "The Cost of Dying: Patients' Last Two Months of Life Cost Medicare $50 Billion Last Year; Is There a Better Way?" *60 Minutes.* November 19. http://www.cbsnews.com/news/the-cost-of-dying/.

Ali, Nadia. 2015. *Medscape.* December 3. Accessed August 8, 2019. https://emedicine.medscape.com/article/2096163-overview.

American Society of Clinical Oncology (ASCO). 2005-2016. "Side Effects of Chemotherapy." *Cancer.net.* Accessed June 7, 2016. http://www.cancer.net/navigating-cancer-care/how-cancer-treated/chemotherapy/side-effects-chemotherapy.

Arenella, Sheryl. n.d. "Coma and Persistent Vegetative State: An Exploration of Terms." *American Hospice Foundation.* https://americanhospice.org/caregiving/coma-and-persistent-vegetative-state-an-exploration-of-terms/.

Bagshow, Robert, Robert C McDermid, and M Sean. 2009. *BioMed Central.* February 12. http://peh-med.biomedcentral.com/articles/10.1186/1747-5341-4-3.

Baile, Walter F. 2000. "A Six-Step Protocol for Delivering Bad News: Application to the Patient with Cancer." *The Oncologist: The Official Jounal of the Society for Translational*

Oncology. June 12. Accessed June 12, 2016. http://theoncologist.alphamedpress.org/content/5/4/302.full.

Balaban, Richard B. 2000. "A Physician's Guide to Talking About End-of-Life Care." *The National Center for Biotechnology Information (NCBI) - J Gen Intern Med. 2000 Mar; 15(3): 195–200.* March 15. http://www.ncbi.nlm.nih.gov/pmc/articles/PMC1495357/.

Breslow, Jason M. 2015. "Prolonging Life or Prolonging Death? Two Doctors on Caring for the Critically Sick." *PBS/Frontline.* February 13. http://www.pbs.org/wgbh/frontline/article/prolonging-life-or-prolonging-death-two-doctors-on-caring-for-the-critically-sick/.

Brody, Jane E. 2009. "End-of-Life Issues Need to Be Addressed." *The New York Times.* August 17. http://www.nytimes.com/2009/08/18/health/18brod.html?_r=0.

Brown-Saltzman, Katherine et al. 2010. "An Intervention to Improve Respiratory Th." *Respiratory Care* 55 (7): 858. Accessed September 14, 2019. https://pdfs.semanticscholar.org/0670/98ed2faf87d4d4fcd772d5d7c1e833060805.pdf.

Center to Advance Palliative Care. 2014. *What Is Palliative Chemotherapy?* March. Accessed June 30, 2017. https://getpalliativecare.org/what-is-palliative-chemotherapy/.

Chandler, Jones. 2019. *Coping with Death and Dying.* February. Accessed September 14, 2019. https://www.researchgate.net/publication/3320 61890_Coping_with_Death_and_Dying.

Christine Cowgill, MS, CRC. 2013. *Urgent Need for Better End-of-Life Training.* June 25. Accessed September 14, 2019. https://www.todaysgeriatricmedicine.com/news /ex_062613.shtml.

Cline, Austin. 2016. "Terri Schiavo's Medical Facts & History." *About.com.* http://atheism.about.com/od/terrischiavonews/a /facts.htm.

Cole, Nicki Lisa. 2015. *Collective Consciousness Defined.* December 29. Accessed February 13, 2017. http://sociology.about.com/od/C_Index/fl/Colle ctive-Consciousness-Defined.htm.

Dasta, Jf, TP McLaughlin, SH Mody, and CT Piech. 2005. "PubMed.org." *US National Library of Medicine National Institutes of Health.* June. http://www.ncbi.nlm.nih.gov/pubmed/1594234 2.

2012. "Definition of Catheter - hemodialysis." *MedicineNet.com.* June 14. http://www.medicinenet.com/script/main/art.as p?articlekey=23012.

Descartes, Rene. 2003. *Meditations and Other Metaphysical Writings.* 2003. Translated by Desmond M. Clarke. London: Penguin Books Ltd. Accessed December 01, 2016.

Drane, James F. 2002. "Honesty in Medicine: should doctors tell the truth?" *Centro Interdisciplinario de Estudios en Bioetica.* Accessed June 10, 20116. http://www.uchile.cl/portal/investigacion/centro-interdisciplinario-de-estudios-en-bioetica/publicaciones/76983/honesty-in-medicine-should-doctors-tell-the-truth.

Duda, Marianne, MS, RDN, LDN, CNSC Clinical Nutritionist. 2017. "Artificial Nutrition and Hydration." 5. Accessed June 6, 2017.

Dunn, Hank. 2016. *Hard Choices for Loving People: CPR, Feeding Tubes, Comfort Measures, and the Patient with a Serious Illness.* Naples, Florida: Quality of Life Publishing.

Dyck, Janice Van. 2011. "Go Ahead. It's Okay to Die." *The Huffington Post.* September 16. Accessed June 15, 206. http://www.huffingtonpost.com/janice-van-dyck/letting-go-to-death_b_962696.html.

Fitzpatrick, Jeanne and Eileen M. Fitzpatrick. 2010. *A Better Way of Dying: How to Make the Best Choices at the End of Life.* New York, New York: Penguin Group (USA). Accessed January 31, 2016.

Fitzpatrick, Jeanne, and Eileen M. Fitzpatrick. 2010. *A Better Way of Dying: How to Make the Best Choices at the End of Life.* New York, New York: Penguin Group (USA). Accessed January 31, 2017.

FloridaHealthFinder.gov. n.d. "Health Care Advance Directives." *FloridaHealthFinder.gov.*

Accessed May 28, 2017.
http://www.floridahealthfinder.gov/reports-
guides/advance-directives.aspx.

Gawande, Atul. 2014. *What doctors don't learn about
death and dying.* October 31. Accessed March
22, 2017. http://ideas.ted.com/death-and-the-
missing-piece-of-medical-school/.

Gawande, Atul,. 2014. "Being Mortal: Medicine and
What Matters in the End." New York, New
York: Metropolitan Books: Henry Holt and
Company, LLC. 154.

Goldthrite, Sarah. 2016. *Death Education for
Professions: DOA?* July 29. Accessed
September 14, 2019.
http://nursing.buffalo.edu/news-
events/latest_news.host.html/content/shared/nu
rsing/articles/academic_articles/death-
education.detail.html.

Grady, Denise. 2005. "The Hard Facts Behind a
Heartbreaking Case." *New York Times: Week
in Review.* June 19.
http://www.nytimes.com/2005/06/19/weekinre
view/the-hard-facts-behind-a-heartbreaking-
case.html?_r=0.

GreekGods.Org - Mythology of Ancient Greece. 2016.
"Eos (Aurora, Dawn)." *GreekGods.org.*
http://www.greek-gods.org/titans/eos.php.

Guadagnino, Christopher. 2012. "Patient Satisfaction
Critical to Hospital Value-Based Purchasing
Program." *The Hospitalist: An official
publication of the Society of Hospital Medicine.*
October 1. Accessed June 15, 2016.

http://www.the-hospitalist.org/article/patient-satisfaction-critical-to-hospital-value-based-purchasing-program/?singlepage=1.

Heilweil, Rebecca. 2016. *Learning Loss: Nursing students cope with patient death.* February 24. Accessed September 14, 2019. https://www.thedp.com/article/2016/02/learning-loss-nursing-students-cope-with-patient-death.

Jason, Zachary. 2018. *The Vigil.* February 18. Accessed September 14, 2019. https://www.bc.edu/bc-web/schools/cson/cson-news/TheVigil.html.

Joss, Fiona Cocquer and Nerida. 2016. *Compassion Fatigue among Healthcare, Emergency and Community Service Workers: A Systematic Review.* June 22. Accessed September 14, 2019. https://www.mdpi.com/1660-4601/13/6/618.

Karnes, Barbara. 2014. *Gone From My Sight: The Dying Experience.* Vancouver, Washington: Barbara Karnes Books, Inc. Accessed February 1, 2017.

Kaufman, Sharon R. 2005. *...and a time to die: How American Hospitals Shape the End of Life.* Chicago, Illinois: The University of Chicago Press. Accessed January 31, 2016.

Kaufman, Sharon R. 2005. *...and a time to die: How American Hospitals Shape the End of Life.* Chicago, Illinois: The University of Chicago Press. Accessed January 30, 2017.

Kaufman, Sharon, R. 2005. *...and a time to die: How American Hospitals Shape the End of Life.* Chicago, Illinois: The University of Chicago Press. Accessed January 31, 2017.

Kelley, Maggie Callanan and Patricia. 1992. *Final Gifts: Understanding the Special Awareness, Needs, and Communications of the Dying.* New York, New York: Simon & Shuster Paperbacks: A Division of Simon & Schuster, Inc. Accessed February 1, 2017.

Kelm, Diana J, Jared T. Perrin, Rodrigo Cartin-Ceba, Ognjen Gajic, Louis Schenck, and Cassie C. Kennedy. 2015. "Fluid Overload in Patients with Severe Sepsis and Septic Shock Treated with Early-Goal Directed Therapy is Associated with Increased Acute Need for Fluid-Related Medical Interventions and Hospital Death." *Shock* (National Center for Biotechnology Information, U.S. National Library of Medicine) 43 (1): 68-73. Accessed July 12, 2017. https://www.ncbi.nlm.nih.gov/pmc/articles/PMC4269557/.

Kenen, Joanne. 2015. "The ACA and patient satisfaction: Does it improve care?" *Association of Healthcare Journalists: Center for Excellence in Healthcare Journalism.* May 6. Accessed June 15, 2016. http://healthjournalism.org/blog/2015/05/the-aca-and-patient-satisfaction-does-it-improve-care/.

Knowles, Megan. 2018. "Majority of patients misjudge CPR success rates: 4 things to know." *Becker's Healthcare.* February 27. Accessed November 27, 2019. https://www.beckershospitalreview.com/qualit y/majority-of-patients-misjudge-cpr-success-rates-4-things-to-know.html.

Landau, Elizabeth. 2013. "When 'life support' is really 'death support'." *CNN.* December 29. http://www.cnn.com/2013/12/28/health/life-support-ethics/.

Lasagna, Luis. 2016. "Bioethics: Hippocratic Oath, Modern Version." *John Hopkins Sheridan Libraries and University Museums.* June 1. http://guides.library.jhu.edu/c.php?g=202502& p=1335759.

Leigh. 2019. *AED.US.* Accessed August 7, 2019. http://www.aed.us/blog/aed-info/the-american-heart-association-changes-their-guidelines-for-2019/.

L'Hommedieu Stankus, Jennifer. 2009. "An Attorney's Thoughts on Truth Telling." *American College of Emergency Physicians.* June. Accessed May 22, 2017. https://www.acep.org/clinical---practice-management/an-attorney-s-thoughts-on-truth-telling/.

2011. "Life Support Choices." *Society of Critical Care Medicine.* http://www.myicucare.org/Adult-Support/Pages/Life-Support-Choices.aspx.

Lowry, Fran. 2013. "Do Patients Need to Know They Are Terminally Ill?" *Medscape.* May 02.

Accessed May 2016.
http://www.medscape.com/viewarticle/803535.

Mahan, K. 2019. *Death and Dying: Tools to Help
Respiratory Therapists Handle Frequent
Exposure to End of Life Care.* Accessed
September 14, 2019.
https://www.ncbi.nlm.nih.gov/pubmed/308268
34.

Mamede, S, and HG Schmidt. 2014. *PubMed: U.S.
National Library of Medicine - National
Institutes of Health.* January.
http://www.ncbi.nlm.nih.gov/pubmed/2433011
5.

McConnell, Kristin. 2012. "Diary of an intensive-care
nurse." *New York Post.* December 9.
http://nypost.com/2012/12/09/diary-of-an-
intensive-care-nurse/.

McEntyre, Marilyn Chandler. 2015. *A Long Letting
Go: Meditations on losing someone you love.*
Grand Rapids, Michigan: Wm. B. Eerdmans
Publishing Co. Accessed December 01, 2016.

Meier, Diane E. 2006. "AMA Journal of Ethics®
Volume 8, Number 9: 564-570." *America
Medical Association: Journal of Ethics.*
September. Accessed June 11, 2016.
http://journalofethics.ama-
assn.org/2006/09/ccas2-0609.html.

Michael P Donahoe, M.D. 2012. "Current Venues of
Care and Related Costs for the Chronically
Critically Ill." 57 (6): 868. Accessed March 22,
2017. http://rc.rcjournal.com/content/57/6/867.

Moller, David Wendell. 2000. *Life's End: Technocratic Dying In An Age Of Spiritual Yearning.* New York , New York: Baywood Publishing Co., Inc. Accessed February 1, 2017.

Nuland, Sherwin B. 1995. *How We Die: Reflections of Life's Final Chapter.* New York, New York: First Vintage Books Edition. Accessed January 31, 2017.

O'Kelly, Clarissa de Pentheny, Catherine Urch, and Edwina A Brown. 2011. "Nephrology Dialysis Transplantation." *Oxford Jounals.* September 26. Accessed June 7, 2016. http://ndt.oxfordjournals.org/content/26/12/3838.full.

Online Sunshine - Official Internet Site of the Florida Legislature. 2016. "Chapter 709." *The 2016 Florida Statutes.* Accessed May 28, 2017. http://www.leg.state.fl.us/Statutes/index.cfm?App_mode=Display_Statute&URL=0700-0799/0709/0709.html.

Ray, John. 2019. *Wikipedia: The Free Encyclopedia.* November 17. Accessed January 09, 2020. https://en.wikipedia.org/wiki/The_road_to_hell_is_paved_with_good_intentions.

Rinpoche, Sogyal. 2002. *The Tibetan Book of Living And Dying.* New York, New York: HaperCollins Publishers. Accessed February 8, 2017.

Rosenberg, Yuval. 2012. "Out-of-Pocket Medical Costs Threaten Seniors ." *The Fiscan Times.* September 10.

http://www.thefiscaltimes.com/Articles/2012/0
9/10/Out-of-Pocket-Medical-Costs-Threaten-
Seniors.

Sanchez, Ray. 2016. "California family given more
time, can keep son on ventilator." *CNN.* May
13.
http://www.cnn.com/2016/05/12/health/califor
nia-israel-stinson-case/.

SCAFoundation . 2018. *Sudden Cardiac Arrest
Foundation.* February 1. Accessed August 7,
2019. https://www.sca-aware.org/sca-
news/aha-releases-latest-statistics-on-sudden-
cardiac-arrest.

Schneider, Patrick A., et al. 1992. "In-Hospital
Cardiopulmonary Resuscitation: A 30 Year
Review." October 16.
http://www.jabfm.org/content/6/2/91.full.pdf.

Span, Paula. 2012. "How Successful is CPR in Older
Patients?" *The New Old Age: Caring and
Coping.* August 9.
http://newoldage.blogs.nytimes.com/2012/08/0
9/how-successful-is-cpr-in-older-
patients/?_r=0.

Stix, Madeleine,. 2013. "Un-extraordinary measures:
Stats show CPR often falls flat." *CNN Health.*
July 10.
http://www.cnn.com/2013/07/10/health/cpr-
lifesaving-stats/.

Stix, Madeleine. 2013. *Un-extraordinary measures:
Stats show CPR often falls flat.* July 20.
Accessed March 2017, 2017.

http://www.cnn.com/2013/07/10/health/cpr-lifesaving-stats/.

Strickland, Shawna L. 2016. "Respiratory Therapists' Involvement in End-of-Life Discussions: Stepping Up to the Plate." *Respiratory Care* 61 (7): 992. Accessed September 14, 2019. http://rc.rcjournal.com/content/61/7/992.

Tremmel, William Calloley,. 1976. *Religion: What Is It?* Holt, Rinehart and Winston. Accessed December 01, 2016.

Tremmel, William Calloley:. 1976. *Religion: What Is It?* Holt, Rinehart and Winston. Accessed November 30, 2016.

Tremmel, William, Calloley:. 1976. *Religion - What Is It?* Tampa, Florida: Holt, Rinehart and Winston.

West's Encyclopedia of American Law, edition 2. S.v. 2016. "The Free Dictionary." *"Death and Dying".* May 27. http://legal-dictionary.thefreedictionary.com/Death+and+Dying.

Whoriskey, Peter. 2014. "'Warehouses for the dying': Are we prolonging life or prolonging death?" *The Washington Post.* December 14. https://www.washingtonpost.com/news/storyline/wp/2014/12/12/warehouses-for-the-dying-are-we-prolonging-life-or-prolonging-death/.

Williams-Murphy, Monica and Kristan Murphy. 2011. *It's Ok To Die.* MKN, LLC. Accessed February 1, 2017.

Wolcott, Harry. 2008. "Educational Anthropology." *IAE-Pedia.* November. Accessed November 07, 2016. http://iae-pedia.org/Educational_Anthropology.

Wolcott, Harry F. 1991. "Propriospect and the Acquisition of Culture." *Anthropology and Education Quarterly.* September. Accessed June 7, 2016. http://www.jstor.org/stable/3195765?seq=1#page_scan_tab_contents.

Wright, Alexi A., Baohui Zhang, and Alaka Ray. 2008. "Associations Between End-of-Life Discussions, Patient Mental Health, Medical Care Near Death, and Caregiver Bereavement Adjustment." *JAMA: The Journal of the American Medical Association.* October 8. Accessed June 10, 2016. http://jama.jamanetwork.com/article.aspx?articleid=182700.

Yang, Maria. 2013. "http://www.kevinmd.com/blog/2013/02/physicians-tend-decline-cpr-heroic-measures.html." *KevinMd.com.* February 22. http://www.kevinmd.com/blog/2013/02/physicians-tend-decline-cpr-heroic-measures.html.

Yi-Bin, Chen. 2014. *NIH - U.S. National Library of Medicine - Medline Plus.* May 29. Accessed June 7, 2016. https://www.nlm.nih.gov/medlineplus/ency/article/001086.htm.

Youngson, Robert M. 2016. "Pacemakers." *The Free Dictionary.* May 13. http://medical-dictionary.thefreedictionary.com/pacemakers .

Cʒ ꙮ

Index

☙ ❧

I would feel more optimistic about a bright future for man if he spent less time proving that he can outwit Nature and more time tasting her sweetness and respecting her seniority.

E. B. White

About the Author

Enrique is a peaceful individual. His calm demeanor serves as a fountain for the many expressions that bring balance into his life. He is cautious and adventurous, serious and lighthearted, cerebral and intuitive, realistic and spiritual. His wife will tell you that he is enigmatic and unconventional. This is the author in a nutshell

Flashback:

Enrique's inquisitive nature became evident at a very young age as he thrust himself into deep philosophical conversations with his father regarding science, spirituality, religion and metaphysical matters. He will tell you that no topic was off-limits, all he had to do was ask.

Eventually, Enrique pursued diverse studies in pre-med and became a respiratory therapist in 1973. In the early 1980s, he earned a degree in anthropology from the University of South Florida, Tampa. During his anthropological training, two focal points of attraction summoned him: religion and medical anthropology. His educational path continued to draw him to the empirical sciences, and social and behavioral studies. Throughout his years as a practicing respiratory therapist, Enrique continued to study religion and spirituality from a cross-cultural perspective.

In the early 1990s, he accepted the position of Director of Respiratory Care and Pulmonary Rehabilitation at the former Transitional Hospital in Tampa, Florida, but eventually realized that the position distanced him from the hands-on patient care that he preferred. So, he resigned with a purpose.

Enrique's resignation from directorship afforded a sabbatical from the traditional health care system and allowed him to pursue further studies in the field of alternative healing methods such as the effects of sound, pranic healing, auric healing, and various other forms of energy and spiritual work.

In 1996, he became an Usui Shiki Ryoho Reiki Master and a Karuna® Reiki Master and began teaching Reiki Certification Classes under the name, *The Illuminators* in St. Petersburg, Florida. His curriculum included classes on other alternative healing methods, and his teaching platform provided an opportunity to practice spiritual counseling. Enrique went on to earn certifications in Reflexology and Hypnotherapy and became a Certified Chromotherapist, Aura Therapist, Sound Therapist, and Chakra Therapist.

Within a year after his nearing-death experience in 2001, he returned to the healthcare field, but this time, with an entirely different perspective. He recognized the need to integrate holistic practices into Western therapies treating the body, mind, and spirit. Throughout his career of 45 years, his primary area of expertise was caring for critically ill patients and their loved ones. With his renewed vigor and conviction, he successfully melded the Western and Eastern philosophies of patient care into his respiratory care practice until his retirement in 2018.

During his free time, Enrique enjoys playing the tumbadoras, bongos, and guitar. Singing karaoke and dancing with his wife are also favorite pastimes and other creative interests spill over into oil painting, graphic art and photography. None of these things would surprise anyone who knows him and his family since he comes from a long line of talented and gifted artists, musicians and educators.

❖

As he continues to write, his wife asked him,

Why are you finally writing these books?

Engaged in a deep conversation with his keyboard, Enrique paused, raised his eyes over the rim of his round, black-wire glasses, and with a gentle smile said softly and without hesitation,

It's time.

Other Books by the Author

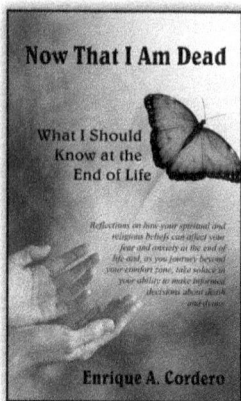

Unlike the author's first book, *It's Hard to Die!,* which focuses on the practical and clinical aspects of the dying process, his second book, *Now That I Am Dead*, presents the subject from a metaphysical and transcendental approach. It addresses issues that impact the mental, emotional, and spiritual dimensions of the dying person, their family, and friends.

It is difficult to step outside our comfort zone, our place of refuge, that little corner in our minds that offers solitude and protection from the unfamiliar. Our comfort zone is our reality, and we protect it from intrusion, especially when it comes to thoughts of death and dying.

If you or a loved one are facing end-of-life issues, this book may help to alleviate the uncertainties and anguish felt during this most heart-rending time. As distressing questions and situations arise, you may be forced to make difficult decisions regarding some various issues:

- Am I playing God?
- Letting go or hanging on
- What happens during the dying process?
- Fear of dying

- Grief and bereavement
- Funeral? Burial? Cremation?
- Being at peace with your religious and spiritual beliefs
- What happens after death?

Perhaps embracing new ideas will open our minds and hearts to a myriad of possibilities. A deeper understanding of the viewpoints of other religions, cultures, and ethnicities will help us become more understanding, compassionate, and respectful of the needs and wishes of the dying person.

Are you ready to journey beyond your comfort zone?

❖

Contact the Author

Email: enrique@eacordero.com
Website: https://www.eacordero.com
Follow: Twitter, Instagram, and Facebook